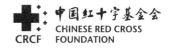

中国红十字基金会
CHINESE RED CROSS
FOUNDATION

CRCF

百年程氏传承系列

U0267242

程氏耳穴应用健康卡册

（中英双语版）

Chengs Auricular Point Health Handbook

（Bilingual Edition）

编　著　程红锋　程　凯

英文审校　丁文静

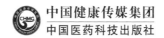

中国健康传媒集团

中国医药科技出版社

内 容 提 要

　　本书是在国医大师程莘农院士学术思想指导下，程氏传承人结合多年耳穴临床经验总结编著而成，主要介绍了标准耳穴及程氏耳穴的临床特色应用，效果显著，应用简单。本书主要包括标准耳穴、经验耳穴、常见疾病耳穴处方应用图卡三部分，图文并茂，简明直观，实用性强，并配有英文翻译，非常适合中医临床医师、中医院校学生、赴外交流从业的专业人员和广大中外中医爱好者等阅读参考。

图书在版编目（CIP）数据

　　程氏耳穴应用健康卡册：中英双语版 / 程红锋，程凯编著. —北京：中国医药科技出版社，2017.5
　　（百年程氏传承系列）
　　ISBN 978-7-5067-8996-7

　　Ⅰ．①程…　Ⅱ．①程…②程…　Ⅲ．①耳－穴位疗法－汉、英　Ⅳ．① R245.9

　　中国版本图书馆 CIP 数据核字（2017）第 029042 号

美术编辑　陈君杞
版式设计　也　在

出版　**中国健康传媒集团** | 中国医药科技出版社
地址　北京市海淀区文慧园北路甲 22 号
邮编　100082
电话　发行：010 - 62227427　邮购：010 - 62236938
网址　www.cmstp.com
规格　889 × 1194mm ¹⁄₃₂
印张　7 ¼
字数　159 千字
版次　2017 年 5 月第 1 版
印次　2022 年 1 月第 4 次印刷
印刷　北京紫瑞利印刷有限公司
经销　全国各地新华书店
书号　ISBN 978-7-5067-8996-7
定价　**48.00 元**

程红锋

国医大师、中国针灸界泰斗程莘农院士长子。程氏针灸第三代传承人。"大诚中医"创始人之一。中国中医科学院退休专家，中国针灸学会耳穴诊治专业委员会委员，香港耳针学会学术顾问。

行医40余载，承家学，纳百家，更潜心研究耳穴，创"程氏疗法"。擅长：使用耳穴治疗甲状腺相关疾病、失眠、戒断综合征、头痛、三叉神经痛及莫名疼痛；运用梅花针治疗青少年近视、远视，儿童弱视，疲劳综合征，面部痤疮，黄褐斑等。

Cheng Hongfeng

The first born son of academician Cheng Xinnong, TCM Master and the most prominent acdemic figure in Chinese Acupuncture. The third generation knowledge inheritor of Chengs Acupuncture. One of the founders of Dacheng TCM. A retired expert of the China Academy of Chinese Medical Sciences, a commissioner of the Auricular Point Therapy Committee of the China Association of Acupuncture and Moxibustion, a consultant for the HK Institute of Auricular Point Therapy.

He has been practicing medicine for more than 40 years. Having learnt directly from his father and the family legacy, absorbed good knowledge and skills from other acupuncture disciplines, he developed an expertise in auricular point therapy and developed "Chengs Approach" of treatment in his practice. He specializes in applying auricular point therapy in treating thyroid related diseases, insomnia, headache, prosopalgia and pains without definite diagnosis, as well as withdrawal syndrome. He is also known for his plum-blossom needle therapy of treating teenage hyperopia, myopia and amblyopia, fatigue, facial acne, chloasma, as so on.

程凯

国医大师、中国针灸界泰斗程莘农院士长孙。中国针灸学会耳穴诊治专业委员会主任委员、国家中医药管理局针灸学重点学科后备学科带头人、中国科协穴位保健首席科学普及专家、中国针灸学会腧穴分会副主任委员、中国针灸学会流派传承与研究专业委员会副主任委员、中国中医药信息研究会养生分会副会长。

中国医师协会养生专业委员会常务理事、世界针灸学会联合会针灸非物质文化遗产传承工作委员会执行委员、世界中医药学会联合会康复保健专业委员会常务理事、北京市针灸学会现代针灸研究专业委员会理事、北京市针灸学会现代针灸研究专业委员会委员。

Cheng Kai

The first born grandson of academician Cheng Xinnong TCM Master and the most prominent authority figure in Chinese Acupuncture. Supervisory commissioner of the Expert Committee of Auricular Point Therapy of the China Institute of Acupuncture and Moxibustion, an academic leader of the auxiliary priority field of research of the State Administration of TCM, chief science officer of acupoint health for the China Association of Science and Technology, deputy supervisory commissioner of Acupoint Committee of the China Association of Acupuncture and Moxibustion, deputy supervisory commissioner of the Expert Committee of School Inheritance and Research of the China Association of Acupuncture and Moxibustion, deputy chairman of the Health Sub-Committee of the China Information Institute of TCM.

Executive director of the Health Expert Committee of the Chinese Medical Doctor Association, executive commissioner of the Acupuncture Intangible Cultural Heritage Committee of the World Federation of Acupuncture-Moxibustion Societies, executive director of the Rehabilitation and Health Expert Committee of the World Federation of Chinese Medicine, commissioner for the Modern Acupuncture Research Expert Committee of the Beijing Association of Acupuncture and Moxibustion.

中国红十字基金会

　　中国红十字基金会（简称"中国红基会"），是全国性公募基金会，国家"5A级基金会"。坚守红十字运动的七项基本原则：人道、公正、中立、独立、志愿服务、统一和普遍。宗旨：弘扬人道、博爱、奉献的红十字精神，致力于改善人的生存状况和发展境况，保护人的生命与健康，促进世界和平与社会进步。

　　中国红基会公益项目以"红十字天使计划"为核心，由健康干预、救灾赈济、教育促进和社区支持四个部分组成，包括贫困重症（白血病、先天性心脏病、唇腭裂、再生障碍性贫血等）儿童医疗救助、乡村卫生院（站）及乡村博爱学校援建、乡村医生及乡村教师培训、灾害及贫困地区博爱家园援建、景区红十字救护站援建等子项目。

The Chinese Red Cross Foundation (CRCF)

CRCF is a national public fundraising organization registered through the Ministry of Civil Affairs. CRCF is ranked as 5A, the top rank, non-profit organizations in China. CRCF sticks to the 7 fundamental principles of the Red Cross and Red Crescent Movement: humanity, impartiality, neutrality, independence, voluntary service, unity and universality. CRCF carries forward the Red Cross spirit of humanity, love and dedication, and commits itself to improving the situation of human living and development, protection of human life and health, and promoting world peace and social progress.

CRCF projects, with "Red Cross Angel Program" as the core, range over health interventions, disaster relief, education and community support, including sub-projects such as medical aid for childen in poverty who suffered severe diseases (leukemia, congenital heart disease, cleft lip and palate, aplastic anemia), construction aid for rural schools and rural medical stations, doctor and teacher training programmes in rural areas, disaster relief in affected and impoverished areas, red cross first-aid stations in tourist attractions.

前　言

从小看父亲用小小耳穴治病，多有奇效。

长大了才知道，耳穴疗法是一种绿色、安全的非药物全息疗法，操作简便，对疼痛、失眠、甲状腺疾病、高血压、糖尿病等多种疾病疗效确切，在快速缓解症状、减少药物用量、辅助或替代常规治疗方面有独特的优势，因此在临床中有很广阔的应用前景。但是，由于近年来对耳穴的推广应用做得很不够，以至于很多医生在临床上不会取耳穴，不会用耳穴处方治疗，广大患者亦不知耳穴的神奇作用。

家父程红锋，曾任中国针灸学会耳穴诊治专业委员会委员、香港耳针学会学术顾问，他潜心研究耳穴几十年，积累了丰富的处方经验，10余年前，我协助父亲将这些耳穴处方经验汇集成册，编辑出版了《耳穴临床应用图卡》（中英对照）一书，深受欢迎。

2014年底，我接任了中国针灸学会耳穴诊治专业委员会的主任委员，推广耳穴更成为分内之事，遂在家父的指导下，对此书进行了修订整理，在收录了新版国家耳穴标准的基础上，结合百年程氏耳穴应用经验，增加了程氏临床经验耳穴及耳穴处方。

本书以日常实用为目的，通过图卡的形式以及通俗易懂的语言将耳穴及耳穴疗法清晰地展现给读者，并配合各类索引信息以方便查找，适合国内外专业从业人员、中医爱好者以及中医院校学生使用。

希望通过此书能够向大众普及耳穴及耳穴疗法，使之广泛应用于大众日常疾病的预防及治疗。

最后，鸣谢中国红十字基金会资助本书出版。

程凯

2017 年 2 月

Preface

Ever since I was a kid, I've been watching my dad operating on the tiny auricular point to cure diseases. More than often, these treatments have miraculous effects.

It was till later I grew up that I comprehended auricular point therapy as a green, secure, non-medicinal holographic physical therapy. It is easy to operate, proven effective to treat various pains, insomnia, thyroid diseases, high blood pressure, diabetes, etc. And it has unique advantage in relieving syndromes rapidly, reducing medical doses and serving as a great complementary or alternative therapy, therefore it has promising application prospects. However, recent years haven't seen nearly enough promotions for the therapy, as a result, doctors fail to utilize such a great technique nor prescribe appropriate formula to treat patients and the amazing therapeutic effects remain unknown to many.

My father, Cheng Hongfeng, once a member of the Expert Committee of Auricular Point Therapy under China Institute of Acupuncture and Moxibustion, a consultant for the HK Institute of Auricular Point Therapy, has studied the therapy for decades and mounted rich experience in acupoint formula. More than 10 years ago, I assisted him in compiling his acupoint formulas, organizing his theories, thoughts and experiences into words. Hence The *Clinical Figured Cards of Auricular Points* (*Bilingual*

Edition) was complied, published and soon enjoyed great popularity.

By the end of the year 2014, I was appointed supervisory commissioner of the Expert Committee of Auricular Point Therapy of the China Institute of Acupuncture and Moxibustion, and promoting auricular point therapy has since officially become a responsibility. Under the guidance of my father, I revised and edited the book again. Based on the New National Regulation of the Auricular Point Therapy, combined with hundred years of accumulated experience of Chengs acupuncture, I further added some auricular points discovered, utilized and proven effective in Chengs clinical experience and acupoint formula.

This book is aimed to help with the regular application of the auricular point by demonstrating with memory cards and plain languages to display the points and the therapy vividly. And the readers could find the points they need by using the search index. It is recommended for professionals both domestically and overseas, TCM enthusiasts, TCM students and beginning learners.

I hope this book make auricular point and the therapy thrive, serve an informative and instructive purpose, and facilitate the prevention and treatment of common diseases.

At last, I'd especially want to express my gratitude to the Chinese Red Cross Foundation for their funding of the book.

Cheng Kai

February 2017

程氏耳穴图卡使用方法
（中／英）

Instructions on How to Use Chengs
Auricular Point Memory Card
（Bilingual Edition）

1.按照病症索引找到相应的图卡，图卡正中为耳正面图，右下为耳背面图，左下为皮质下区放大图。各图中显示的实心黑点是选用的主穴，空心点是选用的配穴，主穴组成处方，配穴随症加减。

Find the right memory cards according to the Index of Disease and Symptoms. The center of the card is the front view of the ear, the lower right corner is the back view of the ear, and the lower left corner comes the amplified figure of Subcortex Area. Black dots in the figure are the main points, while the hollow dots simplify the supplementary points. Formula consists of main points, and supplementary points are symptomatologically selected in accordance with individual conditions.

2.图中所示的三角形位点表示该穴位在内侧面。

Triangle-shaped points indicate that the points are located on the interior.

3.图中所示的穴位点只是大概穴区范围，临床应用时，要用探棒寻找压痛点后再进行治疗。

The locations of the points on the figures just indicate the approximate locations of the points. For clinical applications, the locations need to be checked by detecting responsive spots for pain.

4.另附数张空白卡作为随记便签，记录个人临床经验。

Some blank cards are attached for users to keep a log of their personal experience.

5.随卡附有标准耳穴和经验耳穴的定位、功能及主治，可供使用者学习参考。

Materials about the location, function and indications of both standard and empirical auricular points are attached for user's reference.

目　录
Contents

标准耳穴定位、功能及主治
Location, Function and Indications of Standard
Auricular Point ···································· 1

经验耳穴
The Empirical Auricular Points ·············53

常见疾病耳穴处方应用图卡
The Auricular Point Formula Memory Card for Common Diseases ··· 63

标准耳穴定位、功能及主治

Location, Function and Indications
of Standard Auricular Point

耳中　erzhong（HX1），ear center

1. 定位 Location　在耳轮脚处，即耳轮 1 区。On the crus of the helix, namely the helix 1.

2. 功能 Function　解痉降逆，止呃止逆，理气祛风止痛。Relax muscular spasm, depress abnormal rising of Qi, relieve hiccup and vomiting, promote blood circulation, dispel the wind and relieve pains.

3. 主治 Indications

（1）膈肌痉挛引起的呃逆、呕吐、嗳气、胸闷、脘痞等。也可以用于其他原因引起的呃逆，如胃肠手术后、肝脾肿大、胃肠神经功能紊乱等疾病引起的呃逆。Hiccup, vomiting, belch, discomfort in the chest, fullness, and discomfort in the stomach caused by diaphragmatic spasm. For instance, the hiccup caused by hepatosplenomegaly, gastrointestinal neurosis or post gastrointestinal surgeries complications.

（2）血虚、血瘀、血热引起的诸症及顽固性皮肤瘙痒症。Various symptoms caused by blood deficiency, blood stasis, blood heat, and obstinate cutaneous pruritus.

（3）内脏的某些出血症，如咳血、咯血、崩漏、皮肤紫癜等。Some visceral haemorrhage, such as coughing blood, hemoptysis, metrorrhagia, peliosis, etc.

直肠　zhichang（HX2），rectum

1. 定位 Location　在耳轮脚棘前上方的耳轮处，即耳轮 2 区。On the anterior tip of the superior crus of the helix, namely the helix 2.

2. 功能 Function　有双向的调节作用，即可通便又能止泻。Take effects of two-way adjustment, promote laxation and alleviate diarrhea.

3. 主治 Indications

（1）内外痔、脱肛、便秘、腹泻。Internal and external hemorrhoid, prolapse of anus, constipation, diarrhea.

（2）慢性结肠炎。Chronic colitis.

（3）老年性大便失禁以及痢疾引起的里急后重等症。Senile incontinence of feces and tenesmus caused by dysentery.

（4）皮肤病、鼻咽部疾病。Dermatoses, rhinopharyngeal diseases.

尿道　niaodao（HX3）, urethra

1. 定位 Location　在直肠上方的耳轮处，即耳轮 3 区。On the helix, superior to the point of the rectum, namely the helix 3.

2. 功能 Function　是治疗尿道疾患的经验穴，有清下焦湿热、解痉止痛的作用。A key empirical point to treat urethral diseases, clear away the heat and dampness in the lower energizer, relieve the muscular spasm, and kill pains.

3. 主治 Indications　尿道疾患。如尿急、尿频、癃闭、石淋、尿路感染、尿失禁、尿道狭窄、阴痒、遗精。Urethral diseases, such as dripping, painful or frequent urination, urinary tract infection, urinary incontinence, urethral stricture, pruritus of the genitals, and spermatorrhea.

注：本穴是诊断泌尿系感染的重要参考穴。是鉴别肾小球肾炎与肾盂肾炎的要穴。肾盂肾炎尿道穴可触及条索样改变、尿道穴触痛，探测尿道穴呈阳性反应，而肾小球肾炎在尿道穴探测时呈阴性。

Notes：This point is a valuable reference point to diagnose the urinary infections. It is a key point to differentiate the glomerulonephritis and nephropyelitis. Regarding the nephropyelitis, cord-like change, tenderness could be detected, showing a positive reactions, while as for the glomerulonephritis, the reaction tend to be negative when the same point is detected.

外生殖器 waishengzhiqi（HX4）, external genitals

1. 定位 Location 在对耳轮下脚前方的耳轮处，即耳轮 4 区。On the inferior of the anterior crus of the antihelix, namely the helix 4.

2. 功能 Function 清泄肝胆湿热，凉血祛风止痒，调节性功能。Clear away the dampness and heat in the liver and gallbladder, clear away the blood heat, dispel wind and arrest itchiness, regulate the sexual function.

3. 主治 Indications 外生殖器疾患。Various diseases of genitals.

（1）阴道炎、龟头炎、睾丸炎、附睾炎、输精管结扎手术后、产妇侧切后的阴器肿痛、不适等症。Vaginitis, balanitis, testitis, epididymitis, genital swelling and pain after vasectomies, episiotomies, etc.

（2）阴囊湿疹、外阴瘙痒、阳痿及腰膝酸软、下肢酸痛、下肢无力。Eczema of scrotum, pruritus vulvae, impotence, aching and lassitude of the waists and knees, aching in the lower limbs.

肛门 gangmen（HX5）, anus

1. 定位 Location 在三角窝前方的耳轮处，即耳轮 5 区。On the helix, anterior to the triangular fossa, namely the helix 5.

2. 功能 Function 清热通便，活血消肿止痛。Clear away the heat, promote laxation, promote blood flow, relieve swelling and pain.

3. 主治 Indications 内外痔、脱肛、肛裂、肛门周围炎、肛门脓肿、痢疾、肠炎、大便失禁。Internal and external hemorrhoid, prolapse of the anus, anal fissure, perianal inflammation, perianal abscess, dysentery, and incontinence.

耳尖 erjian（HX6, 7i），ear apex

1. 定位 Location　在耳廓向前对折的上部尖端处，即耳轮 6、7 区交界处。On the top of the helix, namely on the juncture between helix 6 and helix 7.

2. 功能 Function　清热解毒、平肝息风、凉血止痒、消肿止痛。Clear away the heat, remove toxic substances, calm the liver to stop convulsion, cool the blood and arrest itching, relieve swelling and pain.

3. 主治 Indications

（1）头面五官的各种炎症：如麦粒肿、急性结膜炎、急性咽炎、扁桃体炎、面神经炎等。Various cranio inflammations, such as hordeolum, acute conjunctivitis, acute pharyngitis, tonsillitis, facial neuritis, etc.

（2）高血压、神经衰弱、顽固性失眠。Hypertension, neurasthenia, obstinate insomnia.

（3）急性荨麻疹、湿疹以及各种原因引起的热症、痛症、瘀症及皮肤瘙痒症。Acute urticaria, eczema, fever, pain and blood stasis syndrome and cutaneous pruritus caused by various reasons.

注：本穴点刺放血数滴比针刺或贴压疗效好，对炎症、热症疗效更佳。

Notes：The point promises better effects when utilizing bloodletting technique rather than needling or pressing, especially for inflammation and heat syndrome.

结节 （原肝阳穴）jiejie（HX8），node

1. 定位 Location 在耳轮结节处，即耳轮 8 区。On the tubercle of the helix, namely the helix 8.

2. 功能 Function 清肝解毒、涤火潜阳、疏肝解郁。Clear away the heat in liver, remove toxic substances, subdue the Yang of liver, relieve the depressed liver and regulate the circulation of qi.

3. 主治 Indications

（1）肝阳上亢引起的头痛、眩晕、目赤肿痛。Headache, dizziness, conjunctivitis caused by abnormal rising of liver Yang.

（2）急性、慢性肝炎，单项转氨酶增高及胁肋胀痛。Acute and chronic hepatitis, the high level of simplex transaminase and distending pain in the hypochondriac region.

（3）高血压病。Hypertension.

轮 1 lunyi（HX9），helix 1

定位 Location 在耳轮结节下方的耳轮处，即耳轮 9 区。On the helix, inferior to the tubercle of the helix, namely the helix 9.

轮 2 luner（HX10），helix 2

定位 Location 在轮 1 区下方的耳轮处，即耳轮 10 区。On the helix, inferior to the point of the "Helix 1", namely the helix 10.

轮 3 lunsan（HX11），helix 3

定位 Location 在轮 2 区下方的耳轮处，即耳轮 11 区。

On the helix, inferior to the point of "Helix 2," namely the helix 11.

轮 4　lunsi（HX12），helix 4

1. 定位 Location　在轮 3 区下方的耳轮处，即耳轮 12 区。On the helix, inferior to the point of "Helix 3," namely the helix 12.

2. 功能 Function　轮 1 ~ 轮 4 清热解毒、消炎退肿。Helix 1 to Helix 4 could be applied to clear away heat, remove toxic substances, show effects of antiinflammation, subdue swelling.

3. 主治 Indications　各种热症、炎症，如上呼吸道感染、扁桃体炎、咽喉炎、结膜炎、痤疮感染等。Various inflammation and heat syndrome, such as upper respiratory tract infection, tonsillitis, laryngopharyngitis, conjunctivitis, acne infection.

指　zhi（SF1），finger

1. 定位 Location　在耳舟上方处，即耳舟 1 区。On the superior portion of the scaphoid fossa, namely the scaphoid fossa 1.

2. 功能 Function　活血、祛风、通络、镇痛、消炎。Promote blood circulation, dispel wind, activate the meridians, arrest pain and inflammation.

3. 主治 Indications　指部的各种疼痛、指关节扭挫伤、指关节炎、甲沟炎、指部冻伤、腱鞘炎、偏瘫引起的手指运动不灵、雷诺病。Pain and numbness of the fingers, sprain of the finger joint, paronychia, cold bite on fingers, tenosynovitis, post-hemiplegic dysfunction of fingers, Raynaud disease.

腕　wan（SF2），wrist

1. 定位 Location　在指区的下方处，即耳舟2区。
Inferior to the point of finger, namely the scaphoid fossa 2.

2. 功能 Function　活血、祛风、通络、镇痛、消炎、抗过敏。Promote blood flow, dispel wind, activate the meridians, kill pain, show effects of anti-inflammation and anti-anaphylaxis.

3. 主治 Indications　腕部的痛症，如腕关节扭挫伤、类风湿关节炎、腱鞘炎、过敏性鼻炎、荨麻疹。Wrist pain, such as the sprain of wrist joints, rheumatoid arthritis, tenosynovitis, allergic dermatitis, urticaria.

风溪　fengxi（SF1, 2i），wind stream

1. 定位 Location　在耳轮结节前方，指区与腕区之间，即耳舟1、2区交界处。Anterior to the tubercle, between the point of finger and the point of wrist, namely on the junction between the scaphoid fossa 1 and 2.

2. 功能 Function　有良好的抗过敏作用，能活血祛风、止痒、止咳、平喘。Show positive effects of anti-anaphylaxis, promote blood flow, dispel wind and itchiness, relieve cough and asthma.

3. 主治 Indications　各种过敏性疾病及皮肤瘙痒症，如急慢性荨麻疹、湿疹、神经性皮炎、痤疮、哮喘、过敏性鼻炎、过敏性结肠炎。Various allergic diseases and cutaneous pruritus, such as acute and chronic urticaria, eczema, neurodermatitis, acne, asthma, allergic rhinitis and colitis.

注：临床观察对高血压也有一定的疗效。

Note： Clinical practice also shows certain effects on hypertension.

肘 zhou（SF3），elbow

1. 定位 Location 在腕区的下方处，即耳舟3区。Inferior to the point of wrist, namely the scaphoid fossa 3.

2. 功能 Function 活血、祛风、通络止痛。Promote blood flow, dispel wind, activate meridians and arrest pain.

3. 主治 Indications

（1）肱骨外上髁炎、肘部疼痛、风湿性肘关节炎、肘关节挫伤。Tennis elbow, elbow pain, rheumatic arthritis of elbow joint, sprain of elbow joint.

（2）上肢瘫痪、麻木、疼痛、偏瘫等症。Paralysis, numbness, pain of the upper limbs, hemiparalysis

肩 jian（SF4, SF5），shoulder

1. 定位 Location 在肘区的下方处，即耳舟4、5区。Inferior to the point of elbow, namely the scaphoid fossa 4, 5.

2. 功能 Function 活血、祛风、通络止痛。Promote blood flow, dispel wind, activate meridians, arrest pain.

3. 主治 Indications

（1）肩关节周围炎、肩部疼痛、肱二头肌腱炎、风湿症、肩峰下滑囊炎、肩关节扭伤。Scapulohumeral periarthritis, shoulder pain, biceps tendinitis, rheumatic disease, subacromial bursitis, sprain of shoulder joints.

（2）上肢瘫痪、功能障碍。Paralysis and dysfunction of the upper limbs.

（3）颈椎综合征引起的肩部疼痛。Shoulder pain caused by cervical spondylosis.

锁骨　suogu（SF6）, clavicle

1. 定位 Location　在肩区的下方处，即耳舟6区。Inferior to the point of shoulder, namely the scaphoid fossa 6.

2. 功能 Function　散风、祛湿、镇痛。Dispel wind, clear away dampness, kill pain.

3. 主治 Indications　肩关节周围炎、肩背颈部疼痛、风湿痛、无脉症、落枕。Scapulohumeral periarthritis, shoulder pain, back pain, neck pain, rheumatic pain, pulselessness, and stiff neck.

跟　gen（AH1）, heel

1. 定位 Location　在对耳轮上脚前上部，即对耳轮 1 区。On the superior and anterior portion of the superior crus of the antihelix, namely the antihelix l.

2. 功能 Function　活血、祛风、强筋壮骨、消肿止痛。Promote blood flow, dispel wind, strengthen constitution, relieve swelling and pain.

3. 主治 Indications　足跟外伤、感染、冻伤，跟骨骨刺所引起的疼痛，久行引起的跟骨肿痛，跟腱滑囊炎，肾虚性跟骨痛。Heel injury, heel infection, heel frostbite, pain caused by calcaneal spur, swelling and pain in the calcaneal caused by long term walking, Achilles bursitis, calcaneal pain caused by kidney deficiency.

趾　zhi（AH2）, toe

1. 定位 Location　在耳尖下方的对耳轮上脚后上部，即对耳轮 2 区。On the posterior and superior portion of the superior crus of the antihelix, inferior to the ear apex, namely the antihelix 2.

2. 功能 Function 活血祛风、消炎止痛。Promote blood flow, dispel wind, show effects of antiinflammation and arrest pain.

3. 主治 Indications

（1）各种原因引起的趾关节炎症、痛症及瘙痒症，如趾关节扭、冻伤，掌跖皮肤角化症，脚癣，类风湿关节炎，肢端动脉痉挛症，红斑性肢痛症。Various arthritis, pain and pruritus of the toe joints, such as sprain, cold injury of the toe joints, keratosis palmariset plantaris, tinea pedis, rheumatoid arthritis, Raynaud's disease, erythromelalgia.

（2）脑血管意外后遗症，如足趾活动不灵、功能障碍等症。Sequelae of the cerebrovascular accident, such as dysfunction of the toes and toe joints, etc.

踝 huai（AH3），ankle

1. 定位 Location 在趾、跟区下方，即对耳轮 3 区。Inferior to the point of toe and the point of heel, namely the antihelix 3.

2. 功能 Function 活血通络、消肿止痛。Promote blood flow, dispel wind, relieve swelling and pain.

3. 主治 Indications 各种原因引起的踝关节痛，如踝关节扭伤、踝关节功能障碍、风湿痛、跟腱滑囊炎等。Various pains of the ankle joints, such as sprain of the ankle joint, dysfunction of the ankle joint, pain of rheumatic disease, Achilles bursitis, etc.

膝 xi（AH4），knee

1. 定位 Location 在对耳轮上脚中 1/3 处，即对耳轮 4 区。On the middle one-third of the superior crus of the antihelix, namely the antihelix 4.

2. 功能 Function 祛风胜湿、通络止痛。Dispel wind, clear away dampness, activate meridians and arrest pain.

3. 主治 Indications 各种原因引起的膝关节肿痛、下肢功能障碍等症。如风湿性关节炎、膝关节扭伤、髌骨骨折引起的肿痛，以及膝关节退行性骨关节炎、半月板损伤等症。Various swelling and pain of knee joints and dysfunction of the lower limbs, such as rheumatic arthritis, sprain of the knee joints, the swelling and pain caused by fracture of patella, retrograde osteoarthritis of the knee joint, and meniscus injury, etc.

髋　kuan（AH5）, hip

1. 定位 Location 在对耳轮上脚的下 1/3 处，即对耳轮 5 区。On the inferior one-third of the superior crus of the anti-helix, namely the antihelix 5.

2. 功能 Function 活血祛风、通络止痛。Promote blood flow, dispel wind, activate meridians, and arrest pain.

3. 主治 Indications 髋关节疾患。如髋关节炎、髋关节结核、臀部软组织损伤、腰骶部疼痛。Diseases of the hip joint, such as arthritis and tuberculosis of the hip joint, soft tissue injury of the hip, and the lumbosacral pain.

坐骨神经　zuogushenjing（AH6）, sciatic nerve

1. 定位 Location 在对耳轮下脚的前 2/3 处，即对耳轮 6 区。On the anterior two-thirds of the inferior crus of the anti-helix, namely the antihelix 6.

2. 功能 Function　通经活络、强筋壮骨、消肿止痛。

Activate meridians, strengthen muscles and bones, and relieve swelling and pain.

3. 主治 Indications　坐骨神经痛、坐骨神经炎、下肢痿证、痹证、瘫痪。Sciatica, sciatic neuritis, flaccidity, Bi syndrome, and paralysis of the lower limbs.

交感　jiaogan（AH6a）, sympathesis

1. 定位 Location　在对耳轮下脚前端与耳轮内缘相交处，即对耳轮 6 区前端。On the junction of the anterior area of the inferior crus of the antihelix and the interior side of the helix, namely the anterior area of the antihelix 6.

2. 功能 Function　是止酸要穴，有调节交感神经和副交感神经系统的功能，能缓解平滑肌痉挛和调节血管收缩，对内脏器官有较强的镇痛作用，有抑制腺体分泌的作用。It is the key point to suppress acid, showing effects on regulating the functions of sympathetic nerves and parasympathetic nerves, relieving the smooth muscle spasm, regulating blood vessel contraction, killing pains of the internal organs and suppressing certain glands from secreting.

3. 主治 Indications

（1）自主神经功能紊乱引起的诸症。如失眠、多汗、（内脏器官）神经官能症、性功能异常、心律不齐、心动过速等。A wide variety of diseases and syndromes caused by dysfunction of autonomic nerves, including insomnia, hidrosis, psychoneurosis, sexual disorders, arrhythmia, polycardia, etc.

（2）内脏绞痛。如肠绞痛、胆绞痛、肾绞痛、心绞痛以及胃溃疡、哮喘等症。Intense spasmodic pains of the internal organs, such as the intestinal colic, biliary colic, renal colic, angina, gastric ulcer, asthma, etc.

（3）无脉症、脉管炎、大动脉炎、静脉炎、雷诺病等。Pulselessness, vasculitis, aorto-arteritis, phlebitis, Raynaud disease, etc.

（4）眼科和泌尿系疾病等。Ophthalmological diseases and urinary system diseases, etc.

（5）对腺体有抑制分泌作用，常用于治疗胃酸过多。Suppress secretion in certain glands, usually utilized in treating excessive gastric acid.

（6）为胸、腹外科手术中的耳针麻醉常用穴，可代替阿托品。Serve as anesthetic auricular points in some chest and abdomen surgeries, could replace atropine.

注：因气机紊乱引起的腹胀慎用此穴。

Notes：It is not advised to apply this point in the treatment of abdominal distention caused by Qi disorder.

臀　tun（AH7），buttocks

1. 定位 Location　在对耳轮下脚的后 1/3 处，即对耳轮 7 区。On the posterior one-third of the inferior crus of the antihelix, namely the antihelix 7.

2. 功能 Function　活血祛风、通络止痛。Promote blood flow, dispel wind, activate meridians, arrest pain.

3. 主治 Indications　臀骶部疼痛、坐骨神经痛、腰骶神经根炎、臀部软组织损伤等。Buttocks and sacral pain, sciatica, lumbosacral radiculitis, soft tissue injury of the buttocks.

腹　fu（AH8），abdomen

1. 定位 Location　在对耳轮体前部上 2/5 处，即对耳轮

8 区。On the anterior and superior two-fifths of the anti-helix, namely the antihelix 8.

2. 功 能 Function 通经活络、解痉止痛。Activate meridians, relax muscular spasm, arrest pain.

3. 主治 Indications 各种原因引起的腹痛、腹胀、腹泻、肠鸣、便秘等症。如急慢性胃肠炎、肠结核、便秘、腹部手术后腹肌疼痛以及急性腰扭伤、胃肠功能紊乱、溃疡病、胆石症、痛经、月经不调、产后宫缩痛。Abdominal pain and distension, diarrhea, constipation and other symptoms caused by various reasons. For instance, acute or chronic gastroenteritis, intestinal tuberculosis, constipation, postoperative myocelialgia of abdomen, acute lumbar sprain, gastrointestinal dysfunction, ulcer, gallstones, dysmenorrhea, irregular menstruation, and afterpains.

腰骶椎　yaodizhui（AH9），lumbosacral vertebrae

1. 定 位 Location 在腹区后方，即对耳轮 9 区。Posterior to the point of the abdomen, namely the antihelix 9.

2. 功能 Function 壮腰健肾、活血祛风、通络止痛。Strengthen the bones, reinforce the kidney, promote blood flow, dispel wind, activate meridians and arrest pain.

3. 主治 Indications 各种原因引起的腰骶部疼痛及下肢功能障碍。如腰椎间盘突出症、腰椎肥大、腰骶椎挫伤、腰肌劳损、类风湿关节炎、强直性脊柱炎、骶椎隐裂、腰椎骨质增生、下肢麻木、坐骨神经痛以及慢性肾盂肾炎、肾结石等引起的腰痛、遗尿、尿失禁、小便不利等。Lumbosacral pains and dysfunctions of the lower limbs caused by various reasons, such as prolapse of lumbar intervertebral disc, lumbar hypertrophy, lumbosacral bruise, lumbar muscle strain, rheumatoid arthritis, ankylosing spondylitis, sacral vertebrae subfissure, lumbar vertebrae hyperosteogeny, numbness of the lower limbs, sciatica, lumbar pain, enuresis, urinary incontinence, difficulty in micturition caused by chronic pyelonephritis, calculus of kidney, etc.

胸　xiong（AH10）, chest

1. 定位 Location 　在对耳轮体前部中 2/5 处，即对耳轮 10 区。On the middle and anterior two-fifths of the antihelix, namely the antihelix 10.

2. 功能 Function 　镇痛消炎、宽胸理气。Relieve pain, diminish inflammation, alleviate depression and regulate Qi.

3. 主治 Indications 　冠心病引起的胸痛、胸闷、胸膜炎、肋软骨炎、肋间神经痛、带状疱疹、乳腺炎等。Pectoralgia and chest distress, pleurisy, costalchondritis, intercostal neuralgia, herpes zoster, mastadenitis, and other diseases or symptoms caused by coronary heart diseases.

胸椎　xiongzhui（AH11）, thoracic vertebrae

1. 定位 Location 　在胸区后方，即对耳轮 11 区。Poster-ior to the point of chest, namely the antihelix 11.

2. 功能 Function 　活血祛风、通络止痛。Promote blood flow, dispel wind, activate meridians, arrest pains.

3. 主治 Indications 　胸椎退行性病变、胸椎骨质增生、胸背部疼痛及扭挫伤、背部肌肉劳损、肋间神经痛等。Degeneration of thoracic vertebrae, thoracic vertebrae hyperosteogeny, chest and back pains, chest and back bruises, back muscle strain, intercostal neuralgia, etc.

颈 jing（AH12）, neck

1. 定位 Location 在对耳轮体前部下 1/5 处，即对耳轮 12 区。On the anterior and inferior one-fifth of the antihelix, namely the antihelix 12.

2. 功能 Function 具有镇痛及调节甲状腺功能的作用。function to relieve pain and regulate thyroid function.

3. 主治 Indications 落枕、颈项肿痛、颈部扭伤或挫伤、甲状腺肿、甲状腺功能亢进或甲状腺功能减退等。Stiff neck, swelling and pain of the neck, cervical sprain or bruise, thyroid swelling, hyperthyrosis or hypothyrosis, etc.

注：本穴可疏通上、中、下三焦。

Notes: This point has the function of smoothing tri-jiao（or the three energizers）.

颈椎 jingzhui（AH13）, cervical vertebrae

1. 定位 Location 在颈区后方，即对耳轮 13 区。Posterior to the point of neck, namely the antihelix 13.

2. 功能 Function 活血祛风、强筋壮骨、通络止痛。Promote blood flow, dispel wind, strengthen the muscles and bones, activate the meridians to stop pain.

3. 主治 Indications

（1）颈椎骨质增生及各种原因引起的颈部疼痛、颈项强直、斜颈、落枕。Neck pain, neck rigidity, torticollis, stiff neck caused by cervical vertebrae hyperosteogeny or other reasons.

（2）类风湿关节炎、强直性脊柱炎。Rheumatoid arthritis, ankylosing spondylitis.

（3）上肢痿证、痒症、瘫痪。Atrophy, itchiness, paralysis of the upper limbs.

（4）甲状腺肿及甲状腺功能亢进、肥胖症。Thyroid

enlargement or hyperthyrosis, obesity.

（5）是诊断胸椎骨质增生的重要参考穴。Vital reference point of diagnosing the hyperplasia of thoracic vertebrae.

角窝上　jiaowoshang（TF1），superior triangular fossa

1. 定位 Location　在三角窝前 1/3 的上部，即三角窝 1 区。On the anterior and superior one-third of the triangular fossa, namely the triangular fossa 1.

2. 功能 Function　是降压的经验穴，有补肾调肝、养血安神、祛风止痛的功效。Empirical point to decrease blood pressure, regulate and nourish liver and kidney, nourish blood to calm the mind, dispel wind and pain.

3. 主治 Indications　高血压病、头痛、眩晕。Hypertension, headache, vertigo.

内生殖器　neishengzhiqi（TF2），internal genital

1. 定位 Location　在三角窝前 1/3 的中下部，即三角窝 2 区。On the anterior and inferior one-third of the triangular fossa, namely the triangular fossa 2.

2. 功能 Function　补肾益精、调经止带、消炎止痛。Nourish the jing of kidney, regulate menstruation, diminish inflammation, arrest pain.

3. 主治 Indications

（1）月经不调、痛经、闭经、功能性子宫出血、盆腔炎及带下症。Irregular menstruation, dysmenorrhea, amenia, functional uterine bleeding, pelvic inflammation.

（2）睾丸炎、附睾炎、输精管炎。Orchitis, epididymitis, deferentitis.

（3）阳痿、遗精、前列腺炎、性功能减退症、男性不育症、女性不孕症。Impotence, spermatorrhea, prostatitis, diminished sexual capacity, male and female infertility.

注：此穴有调节子宫和催产的作用。

Note：This point can regulate the womb and function to hasten child delivery.

角窝中　jiaowozhong（TF3）, middle triangular fossa

1. 定位 Location　在三角窝中 1/3 处，即三角窝 3 区。On the middle one-third of the triangular fossa, namely the triangular fossa 3.

2. 功能 Function　具有抗过敏、宽胸理气的作用。Anti-anaphylaxis, alleviate depression and regulate qi.

3. 主治 Indications　支气管哮喘、肺气肿、胸闷、气短。Bronchial asthma, pulmonary emphysema, fullness of the chest, shortness of breath.

神门　shenmen（TF4）, shenmen

1. 定位 Location　在三角窝后 1/3 的上部，即三角窝 4 区。On the superior one-third of the triangular fossa, namely the triangular fossa 4.

2. 功能 Function　是止痛要穴，有镇静安神、解痉止痛、消炎止痒、抗过敏、降血压、平肝息风和抑制胃肠蠕动的作用。A key point to relieve pain. Function to calm the nerve, ease spasm, manage pain, diminish inflammation, arrest itchiness, take effects of antianaphylaxis, lower blood pressure, suppress Liver-upheaval and bowel movement.

3. 主治 Indications

（1）神经衰弱、失眠、多梦、烦躁、精神错乱、癔症及忧郁型精神分裂症。Neurasthenic, sleeplessness, dreaminess, dysphoria, confusion, hysteria, and schizophrenia of depressive type.

（2）头面、五官、内脏、肢体的各种炎症、痛症。如头痛、面痛、牙痛、心绞痛、胆绞痛、胃肠痉挛痛、痛经以及各种面神经炎、神经痛。Various inflammations, pains of craniofacial, five-sense organs, viscera and limbs, such as headache, prosopodynia, toothache, angina pectoris, biliary colic, gastrocolostomy, dysmenorrhea, and various neuritis and neuralgia.

（3）高血压。Hypertension.

（4）过敏性疾病。如急性荨麻疹、药物过敏疹、湿疹、神经性皮炎、支气管哮喘、咳嗽（痰多不宜用），及其他瘙痒症。Allergic diseases, such as acute urticaria, drug allergy, eczema, neurodermatitis, bronchial asthma, cough（whereas unfit in cases of excessive sputum）, and other pruritus.

注：临床观察，因气机紊乱引起的腹胀不要用。

Note：Clinical observation indicates that it is not wise to apply this point for abdominal distension due to qi dysfunction.

盆腔　penqiang（TF5）, pelvis

1. 定位 Location　在三角窝后 1/3 的下部，即三角窝 5 区。On the posterior and inferior one-third of the triangular fossa, namely the triangular fossa 5.

2. 功能 Function　清热利湿、通经活络止痛。Clear away heat and dampness, activate the meridians to stop pain.

3. 主治 Indications　盆腔炎、前列腺炎、附件炎、月经不调、腹胀、下肢部疼痛、小腹疼痛及腰骶部酸痛。Pelvic inflammation, prostatitis, adnexitis, irregular menstruation, abdominal distension, lower limbs pain, lower abdominal pain and pain of lumbosacral region.

外耳　waier（TG1u），external ear

1. 定位 Location　在屏上切迹前方近耳轮部，即耳屏 1 区上缘处。On the tragus, anterior to the notch, above the tragus and close to the helix, namely on the upper edge of the tragus 1.

2. 功能 Function　活血化瘀、祛风止痛、通窍聪耳。Promote blood flow and clear away blood stasis, dispel wind and pain, enhance hearing.

3. 主治 Indications　耳部冻伤及感染，外耳道疖肿，耳聋、耳鸣，链霉素中毒引起的耳聋、听力减退，耳廓神经痛，偏头痛，三叉神经痛，头晕，颈项部疼痛，耳廓皮肤病 等。Auricular infection and cold bite, furuncle of external auditory canal, deafness and tinnitus caused by streptomycin, hypoacusis, auricular neuralgic, migraine, trigeminal neuralgia, dizziness, cervical pain, auricular dermatosis.

屏尖　pingjian（TG1p），apex of tragus

1. 定位 Location　在耳屏游离缘上部尖端，即耳屏 1 区后缘处。On the apex of the free edge of the superior tragus, namely on the posterior edge of the tragus 1.

2. 功能 Function　具有消炎、退热、镇静止痛的作用。Take effects of anti-inflammation, abatement of fever, tranquilize the mind and relieve pain.

2. 主治 Indications　各种原因引起的高热、低热、炎症、疼痛，并可治疗牙痛、斜视等。Various hyperthermia, low fever, inflammation, pain, as well as toothache, strabismus etc.

外鼻　waibi（TG1，2i），external nose

1. 定位 Location　在耳屏外侧面中部，即耳屏 1、2 区之间。The center of the exterior edge of the tragus, namely between the tragus 1 and 2.

2. 功能 Function　清热、活血、止痛。Clear away heat, promote blood flow, stop pain.

3. 主治 Indications　鼻疖肿、酒渣鼻、鼻炎、过敏性鼻炎、鼻部痤疮、鼻塞、鼻衄、鼻前庭炎等。Furuncle of nose, brandy nose, rhinitis, rhinallergosis, acne of nose, nasal obstruction, epistaxis, nasal vestibulitis.

肾上腺　shenshangxian（TG2p），adrenal gland

1. 定位 Location　在耳屏游离缘下部尖端，即耳屏 2 区的后缘处。On the apex of free edge of the the inferior tragus, namely on the posterior edge of the tragus 2.

2. 功能 Function　能调节肾上腺和肾上腺皮质激素的功能。有抗过敏、抗风湿、抗感染、退热的作用。有调节血管舒缩功能、兴奋呼吸中枢、止咳平喘的作用。Coordinate the function of adrenal gland and adrenocortical hormone; take effects of anti-rheumatism, anti-infection, and anti-anaphylaxis; abate fever; adjust the dilation and contraction of the blood vessels; excite apneustic center; relieve coughing and asthma.

3. 主治 Indications

（1）不明原因的高热、低热症及风湿性关节炎、腮腺炎等。Hyperthermia, low fever without a definite diagnosis, rheumatic arthritis, parotitis, etc.

（2）胶原组织疾病、各种炎症、过敏性疾病、哮喘、咳嗽及皮肤瘙痒症。Collagen tissue diseases, inflammations, allergic diseases, asthma, cough and pruritus.

（3）低血压、休克、出血性疾病、血管瘤、脉管炎及无脉症等。Hypertension, shock, hemorrhagic diseases, angioma, angitis, and pulselessness.

（4）配合治疗中毒性休克、过敏性休克、呼吸衰竭及输液反应等。Be associated with practices to treat toxic shock, allergic shock, respiratory failure, transfusion reaction, etc.

注：为诊断癌症的参考穴。

Note：A reference point of diagnosing cancer.

咽喉　yanhou（TG3），pharynx and larynx

1. 定位 Location　在耳屏内侧面上 1/2 处，即耳屏 3 区。On the superior half of the internal side of the tragus, namely the tragus 3.

2. 功能 Function　清热解毒、消炎消肿、化痰利咽。Expel toxin by clearing heat, relieve inflammation, subdue swelling, resolve sputum and clear throat.

3. 主治 Indications　急慢性咽喉炎、扁桃体炎、声嘶失语、悬雍垂水肿、气管炎、支气管炎、支气管哮喘、梅核气。Acute and chronic pharyngitis, tonsillitis, hoarseness, staphyloedema, trachitis, bronchitis, bronchial asthma, globus hystericus.

内鼻　neibi（TG4），internal nose

1. 定位 Location　在耳屏内侧面下 1/2 处，即耳屏 4 区。On the inferior half of the interior side of the tragus, namely the tragus 4.

2. 功能 Function 疏风解表、清脑通窍、消炎止血。 Dispel wind and relieve exterior syndrome, wake up the patient from unconsciousness by clearing away heat, take effects of antiinflammation and stop bleeding.

3. 主治 Indications 鼻部各种疾患，如伤风感冒、鼻塞、各种鼻炎、副鼻窦炎、鼻衄等。 Various diseases of the nose, such as cold, nasal obstruction, various rhinitis, paranasal sinusitis, epistaxis, etc.

屏间前（原目 1 穴）pingjianqian（TG2I），anterior intertragal notch

1. 定位 Location 在屏间切迹前方耳屏最下部，即耳屏 2 区下缘处。 On the most inferior part of the tragus, anterior to the intertragic notch, namely on the inferior edge of the tragus.

2. 功能 Function 清热泻火、活血通络、清脑明目。 Clear away heat, promote blood flow, activate meridians, clear away the heat in brain to brighten eyes.

3. 主治 Indications 肝火上炎引起的目赤肿痛、流泪、眩晕、头痛、急慢性青光眼、虹膜睫状体炎、视网膜炎、视神经萎缩、麦粒肿、近视、远视、散光、弱视等。 Conjunctivitis lacrimation, dizziness, headache, acute and chronic glaucoma, iridocyclitis, retinitis, optic atrophy, hordeolum, myopia, hyperopia, astigmia, amblyopia, and other diseases or symptoms caused by flaming-up of the Liver-fire.

额 e（AT1), forehead

1. 定位 Location 在对耳屏外侧面的前部，即对耳屏 1

区。On the anterior part of the antitragus, namely the antitragus 1.

2. 功能 Function　是健脑的要穴，镇静安神、活络止痛、健脑明目。A key point to strengthen the function of brain, tranquil and allay the excitement, activate the meridians to stop pain, strengthen the function of brain and brighten eyes.

3. 主治 Indications

（1）前头痛、头晕、失眠、多梦、神经衰弱、记忆力减退。Frontal headache, dizziness, insomnia, dreaminess, neurasthenia, hypomnesis.

（2）嗜睡、牙痛、鼻炎、额窦炎、屈光不正及弱视。Lethargy, toothache, rhinitis, frontal sinusitis, ametropia and amblyopia.

屏间后 （原目2穴）pingjianhou（AT1l）, posterior intertragal notch

1. 定位 Location　在屏间切迹后方对耳屏前下部，即对耳屏1区下缘处。On the inferior and anterior portion of the antitragus, posterior to the notch between tragus and antitragus, namely on the inferior edge of the antitragus 1.

2. 功能 Function　清热解毒凉血、益精养血明目。Relieve the heat and toxin, cool the blood, nourish jing and xue, brighten the eyes.

3. 主治 Indications　眼底血管病、急性结合膜炎、麦粒肿、虹膜睫状体炎，还可治因眼疾所致的头痛。Angiosis of eye fundus, acute conjunctivitis, hordeolum, iridocyclitis, headache caused by ophthalmopathy.

颞　nie（AT2），temple

1. 定位 Location　在对耳屏外侧面的中部，即对耳屏 2 区。On the middle of the exterior side of the antitragus, namely the antitragus 2.

2. 功能 Function　疏肝泄胆、镇静止痛、明目止鸣。 Relieve the depressed liver and gallbladder, soothe the liver and gallbladder and regulate the circulation of qi, tranquilize the mind and stop pain, brighten eyes and cure tinnitus.

3. 主治 Indications

（1）偏正头痛、头晕、头昏、嗜睡及由其引起的遗尿。 Migraine, dizziness, lethargy and accompanied enuresis.

（2）眼睛屈光不正、耳鸣、听力减退。Ametropia, tinnitus, hypoacusis.

枕　zhen（AT3），occiput

1. 定位 Location　在对耳屏外侧面的后部，即对耳屏 3 区。On the posterior of the exterior side of the antitragus, namely the antitragus 3.

2. 功能 Function　是止晕的要穴，有清热息风、镇痉安神、止痛、止咳、平喘、止痒、止吐明目的作用。A key point of relieving dizziness, clear away heat and suppress the abnormal liver-wind, allay excitement, stop pain, relieve cough and asthma, dispel itchiness, stop vomiting and brighten eyes.

3. 主治 Indications

（1）脑炎、脑膜炎，脑外伤，脑血管意外引起的抽搐、角弓反张、牙关紧闭、颈项强直等。Cerebritis, meningitis, brain trauma, and convulsion, opisthotonus, trismus, stiff neck caused by cerebrovascular accident.

（2）大脑供血不足引起的头晕、头痛及晕车、晕机、晕船等。Dizziness, headache, and carsickness, seasickness, airsickness caused by cerebral ischemia.

（3）皮层性视力障碍、老年眼花、视物不清以及近视、远视、弱视、白内障等。Cortical visual disturbance, presbyopia, blurring of vision, myopia, hyperopia, amblyopia, cataract, etc.

（4）失眠、多梦及顽固性皮肤瘙痒症。Insomnia, dreaminess, obstinate pruritus.

（5）哮喘、运动病。Asthma, motion sickness.

皮质下　pizhixia（AT4）, subcortex

1. 定位 Location　在对耳屏内侧面，即对耳屏4区。On the interior side of the antitragus, namely the antitragus 4.

2. 功能 Function　有调节大脑皮层的兴奋与抑制的功能，具有益脑安神、消炎止痛、止呕止呃、苏厥救脱的作用。Regulate the function of cerebral cortex excitation or inhibition, nourish the brain and calm the mind, dephlogisticate, dispel pain, relieve hiccup and vomiting, revive yang for resuscitation.

3. 主治 Indications

（1）大脑皮层的兴奋和抑制失调引起的各种病症。如失语、多梦、记忆力下降、神经衰弱等。Diseases caused by dysfunction of the cortex, such as insomnia, dreaminess, hypomnesis, neurasthenia, etc.

（2）消化系统疾病。如消化不良、胃炎、胃及十二指肠球部溃疡、恶心呕吐、腹胀、便秘及肝、胆、胰系疾病。Diseases of digestive system, such as dyspepsia, gastritis, gastroduodenal ulcer, nausea, vomiting, abdominal distension, constipation, as well as hepatic diseases, biliary diseases, and pancreatic diseases.

（3）心血管系统疾病。如高血压、大动脉炎、血栓闭塞性脉管炎、静脉炎、雷诺病、冠心病、心律失常等。Angiocardiopathy diseases, such as hypertension, aortoarteritis, thromboangitis, phlebitis, the Raynaud disease, coronary heart disease, arrhythmia, etc.

（4）顽固性炎症、痛症、呕吐及呃逆。Obstinate inflammation, pain, vomiting and hiccup.

（5）配合治疗中毒性休克及昏厥。Be associated in practice to treat the toxic shock and faint.

对屏尖　duipingjian（AT1, 2, 4i）, apex of antitragus

1. 定位 Location　在对耳屏游离缘的尖端，即对耳屏1、2、4区之交点。On the apex of the free edge of the antitragus, namely the point of intersection among antitragus 1, 2 and 4.

2. 功能 Function　能调节呼吸中枢，具有抗过敏、止咳平喘、消炎止痒的作用。Regulate apneustic center, take effects of anti-anaphylaxis, relieve cough and asthma, dephlogisticate and dispel itchiness.

3. 主治 Indications

（1）呛咳、哮喘、气急、胸闷、呼吸困难等症。Cough, asthma, short breath, oppressed feeling in chest, dyspnea, etc.

（2）腮腺炎、睾丸炎。Parotitis, orchitis.

（3）皮肤瘙痒症、神经性皮炎。Cutaneous pruritus, neurodermatitis.

缘中 yuanzhong（AT2, 3, 4i）, central rim

1. 定位 Location 在对耳屏游离缘上，对屏尖与轮屏切迹之中点处，即对耳屏2、3、4区的交点处。On the free edge of the antitragus, in the middle of the antitragic apex and the the helix notch, namely on the junction among the antitragus 2, 3 and4.

2. 功能 Function 有调节脑垂体功能及镇痉息风、益脑健神之效，还有抗过敏、抗休克、止血的作用。Regulate pituitary function, stop endogenous wind, relieve muscular spasm, nourish the brain, take effects of anti-anaphylaxis and anti-shock, and stop bleeding.

3. 主治 Indications

（1）脑炎后遗症、脑震荡后遗症、大脑发育不全等。Sequelae of encephalitis and cerebral concussion, cerebral dysgenesis, etc.

（2）梅尼埃病。Meniere's disease.

（3）脑垂体功能障碍所引起的休克、呼吸衰竭。Respiratory failure, shock caused by hypophysis dysfunction.

脑干 naogan（AT3, 4i）, brainstem

1. 定位 Location 在屏轮切迹正中凹陷处。In the central cavity of the notch between tragus and helix.

2. 功能 Function 息风止痉、益脑安神，是镇痉良穴。Stop endogenous wind, relieve muscular spasm, replenishing the brain and tranquilizing the mind, a key point of relieving muscular spasm.

3. 主治 Indications 脑膜刺激征。如癫痫、精神分裂症、神经官能症、低热、梅尼埃病、遗尿、过敏性皮炎、头痛等。Meningeal irritation, such as epilepsy, schizophrenia, neurosis, lower fever, Meniere's disease, enuresis, contact dermatitis, headache etc.

口 kou（CO1）, mouth

1. 定位 Location　在耳轮脚下方前 1/3 处，即耳甲 1 区。On the anterior one-third of the concha, under the inferior crus of the antihelix, namely the superior concha 1.

2. 功能 Function　疏风通络、镇静止咳、止痛、消炎解痉、调节胃肠功能。Eliminate wind and activate meridians, relieve muscular spasm, relieve cough and asthma, arrest pain and regulate gastrointestinal function.

3. 主治 Indications　面瘫、戒断综合征、胆囊炎、胆石症、各种疾病引起的口味异常、口腔溃疡、口腔炎、咽喉炎、舌炎、牙周炎、哮喘、咳嗽、失眠、烦躁，还可治疗劳累后腰膝酸痛乏力。Facial paralysis, abstinence syndrome, cholecystitis, cholelithiasis, abnormal taste due to various kinds of diseases, oral ulcer, stomatitis, glossitis, laryngopharyngitis, periodontitis, bronchial asthma, cough, insomnia, irritability, sore pain of lumbar region and knee joints after overwork.

注：此穴有一定的镇静作用，可用于催眠。
Note：This point has sedative function, could be used to induce sleep.

食道 shidao（CO2）, esophagus

1. 定位 Location　在耳轮脚下方中 1/3 处，即耳甲 2 区。On the middle one-third of the concha, which is under the inferior crus of the antihelix, namely the superior concha 2.

2. 功能 Function　是治疗吞咽困难的经验穴。有通利食道、增进食欲、宽胸利膈的功效。An empirical point to treat dysphagia, regulate esophagus, enhance appetite, alleviate depression to regulate qi.

3. 主治 Indications 吞咽困难、食道处痛、食道痉挛、食道炎、胸闷、憋气、呼吸不畅、梅核气、失眠。Dysphagia, esophageal pain, esophageal tuberculosis, esophagitis, chest distress, short breath, hypopnea, globus hystericus, insomnia.

贲门 benmen（CO3）, cardia

1. 定位 Location 在耳轮脚下方后 1/3 处，即耳甲 3 区。 On the posterior one-third of the inferior crus of the helix, namely the superior concha 3.

2. 功能 Function 和胃止痛、缓解痉挛、增进食欲。Regulate stomach to stop pain, relieve spasm, enhance appetite.

3. 主治 Indications 贲门疾患，如贲门痉挛、恶心、呕吐、胸部不适、溃疡病等。Cardial diseases, such as cardiospasm, nausea, vomiting, chest discomfort, ulcer, etc.

胃 wei（CO4）, stomach

1. 定位 Location 在耳轮脚消失处，即耳甲 4 区。On the terminus of the inferior crus of the helix, namely the superior concha 4.

2. 功能 Function 和胃健脾、降逆止呕、解痉止痛、补中益气。Regulate stomach to smooth qi and invigorate spleen, regulate the reversed flow of qi and relieve vomiting, relieve muscular spasm to stop pain, tonify spleen to nourish qi.

3. 主治 Indications

（1）各种胃病：胃炎、胃溃疡、胃脘痛、胃痉挛、胃肠功能紊乱、消化不良。Various gastropathy, such as gastritis, gastric ulcer, epigastralgia, gastrospasm, gastrointestinal dysfunction, dyspepsia.

（2）胃气上逆之症，如：恶心、呕吐。Nausea, vomiting caused by abnormal rising of Stomach-qi.

（3）前头痛、牙痛、失眠等。Frontal headache, toothache, insomnia, etc.

十二指肠　shierzhichang（CO5），duodenum

1. 定位 Location　在耳轮脚及部分耳轮与 AB 线之间的后 1/3 处，即耳甲 5 区。On the posterior one-third of the portion between the inferior crus of the helix and AB line, namely the superior concha 5.

2. 功能 Function　解痉止痛、调节胃肠功能。Relieve spasm and pain, regulate gastrointestinal function.

3. 主治 Indications　十二指肠球部溃疡、胆囊炎、胆石症、幽门痉挛、上腹部疼痛、消化不良、腹胀、泄泻、小儿厌食。Used for duodenal bulbar ulcer, cholecystitis, cholelithiasis, pylorospasm, epigastralgia, dyspepsia, abdominal distension, diarrhea, infantile anorexia.

小肠　xiaochang（CO6），small intestine

1. 定位 Location　在耳轮脚及部分耳轮与 AB 线之间的中 1/3 处，即耳甲 6 区。On the middle one-third of the portion between the superior crus of the helix and the AB line, namely the inferior concha 6.

2. 功能 Function　分清别浊、清热利湿、通便止泻、行气散结、清心降火、镇静安神、调节心律。Separate the clear from the turbid, clear away dampness and heat, promote laxation or relieve diarrhea, promote circulation of qi and remove obstruction, eliminate the heart-fire, tranquilize and allay excitement, regulate heart rhythm.

3. 主治 Indications

（1）消化不良、腹泻、腹胀、胃肠吸收功能障碍引起的消瘦症、十二指肠球部溃疡、肠结核。Dyspepsia, diarrhea, abdominal distension, emaciation caused by dysfunction of gastrointestinal absorption, gastroduodenal ulcer, intestinal tuberculosis.

（2）心动过速、心烦、心律不齐、冠心病。Tachycardia, vexation, arrhythmia, coronary heart disease.

（3）口舌生疮、咽痛等。Aphthae, sore-throat.

（4）小便不利、小便赤。Difficulty in micturition, dark yellow urine.

大肠　dachang（CO7），large intestine

1. 定位 Location　在耳轮脚及部分耳轮与 AB 线之间的前 1/3 处，即耳甲 7 区。On the anterior one-third of the portion between the inferior crus of the helix and the AB line, namely the superior concha 7.

2. 功能 Function　传导糟粕、清热祛风、止咳通便、止泻。Conduct the waste, remove heat to relieve convulsion, relieve cough, facilitate laxation, relieve diarrhea.

3. 主治 Indications

（1）肠功能紊乱、痢疾、肠炎、腹泻、阑尾炎、便秘、大便失禁、肠结核、肠粘连等。Intestinal dysfunction, dysentery, enteritis, diarrhea, constipation, appendicitis, fecal incontinence, intestinal tuberculosis, intestinal adhesion, etc.

（2）咳嗽、气喘、感冒、肺炎等呼吸道疾病，以及皮肤瘙痒、痤疮。Respiratory diseases such as cough, asthma, cold, pneumonia, pruritus and acne.

阑尾　lanwei（CO6, 7i）, appendix

1. 定位 Location　在小肠区和大肠区之间，即耳甲6、7区交界处。Between the point of Large and small intestine, namely on the juncture between superior concha 6 and 7.

2. 功能 Function　是治疗阑尾炎的经验穴。有清热解毒、活血、止痛的作用。A key empirical point to treat appendicitis, expel toxin by clearing away heat, promote blood flow to stop pain.

3. 主治 Indications　急慢性阑尾炎、下腹部疼痛、腹泻。Acute or chronic appendicitis, hypogastralgia, diarrhea.

艇角　tingjiao（CO8）, angle of superior concha

1. 定位 Location　在对耳轮下脚下方前部，即耳甲8区。On the anterior portion of the concha, inferior to the inferior crus of the helix, namely the concha 8.

2. 功能 Function　补肾益精、清热利湿、活血化瘀、消坚散结。Replenish the vital essence by nourishing kidney, eliminate dampness by cooling, promote blood flow to remove blood stasis, eliminate blood stasis to remove abdominal mass.

3. 主治 Indications　前列腺炎、前列腺肥大、尿道炎及男性性功能减退、支气管哮喘、喘息样支气管炎、鼻衄、脑血管疾病、功能性子宫出血。Prostatitis, prostatic hyperplasia, urethritis, male hypogonadism, bronchial asthma, asthmatic bronchitis, epistaxis, cerebrovascular disease, functional uterine bleeding.

膀胱　pangguang（CO9）, bladder

1. 定位 Location　在对耳轮下脚下方中部，即耳甲 9 区。On the middle portion of the concha inferior to the inferior crus of the helix, namely concha 9.

2. 功能 Function　清利湿热、化气行水、通络止痛。Relieve dampness and heat, regulate the circulation of qi and water, activate the meridians to stop pain.

3. 主治 Indications

（1）急性膀胱炎、肾盂肾炎、前列腺炎、夜尿症、尿频、尿急、尿痛、尿失禁等。Acute cystitis, pyelitis, prostatitis, nocturia, frequency of micturition, urgency of urination, urodynia, urinary incontinence, etc.

（2）后头痛、腰脊痛、坐骨神经痛。Backache, pain along spinal column, sciatica.

肾　shen（CO10）, kidney

1. 定位 Location　在对耳轮下脚下方后部，即耳甲 10 区。On the posterior portion of the concha, inferior to the inferior crus of the helix, namely the concha 10.

2. 功能 Function　滋阴壮阳、补肾益精强腰脊、通利水道、明目聪耳、扶正抗衰。Nourish yin and strengthen yang, replenish vital essence of kidney, strengthen the back, regulate fluid passage, improve eyesight and hearing, strengthen the body in resistance against senescence.

3. 主治 Indications

（1）各种慢性虚弱性疾病，如：肾炎、肾盂肾炎、五更泻、腰膝酸软、足跟痛等症。Various chronic and debilitating diseases, such as nephritis, pyelonephritis, diarrhea before dawn, lassitude in loin and legs, pain in the heel, etc.

（2）脑髓不足所致的健忘、头晕、失眠、牙齿松动；类风湿关节炎、骨质增生以及骨关节退行性病变等。Amnesia, dizziness, insomnia, gomphiasis caused by deficiency of brain and spinal marrow; rheumatoid arthritis, hyperosteogeny, osteoarthrosis, etc.

（3）男女生殖系统的病症，如阳痿、遗精、月经不调、不孕不育症等。Reproductive diseases, such as impotence, spermatorrhea, irregular menstruation, infertility, etc.

（4）耳鸣、耳聋、脱发、斑秃等。 Deafness, tinnitus, baldness, alopecia, areata, etc.

（5）各种水液代谢失常所致的疾病，如水肿、小便不利等。Edema, difficulty in micturition, and other diseases or symptoms caused by dysfunction of water metabolism.

（6）由各种慢性虚弱病引起的功能低下症及肾虚泄泻、夜尿过多、遗尿等。Hypofunction, diarrhea due to kidney insufficiency, polyuria at night, and other diseases or symptoms caused by chronic debilitating diseases.

输尿管　shuniaoguan（CO9, 10i），ureter

1. 定位 Location　在肾区与膀胱区之间，即耳甲9、10区交界处。Between the point of kidney and the point of bladder, namely on the juncture between the concha 9 and 10.

2. 功能 Function　清下焦湿热、解痉止痛。Clear away heat and dampness in lower-jiao, relax the spasm to stop pain.

3. 主治 Indications　泌尿系感染、输尿管结石。Urinary

infections, ureterolithiasis.

胰胆　yidan（CO11）, pancreas and gallbladder

1. 定位 Location　在耳甲艇的后上部，即耳甲 11 区。On the posterior and superior portion of the superior concha, namely the concha 11.

2. 功能 Function　疏肝利胆、解痉消炎、通络止痛。Disperse the depressed qi of liver and gallbladder, relieve muscular spasm, antiinflammation, activate the meridians to stop pain.

3. 主治 Indications

（1）胆道疾患：如胆囊炎、胆石症、胆道蛔虫症、口苦、胸胁胀满。Biliary diseases, such as cholecystitis, cholelithiasis, parasitic disease of biliary tract, bitter taste, fullness of hypochondriac region.

（2）急慢性胰腺炎、肝炎、糖尿病、消化不良。Acute or chronic pancreatitis, hepatitis, diabetes mellitus, dyspepsia.

（3）耳聋、耳鸣、偏头痛、颈项强直、失眠多梦等。Deafness, tinnitus, migraine, stiff neck, insomnia, dreaminess, etc.

肝　gan（CO12）, liver

1. 定位 Location　在耳甲艇的后下部，即耳甲 12 区。On the posterior and inferior portion of the superior concha, namely the concha 12.

2. 功能 Function　疏肝理气、活血化瘀、疏风开窍、舒筋止疼、祛风除痰、益目。Alleviate the depressed liver, soothe the liver and regulate the circulation of qi, promote the blood circulation and remove blood stasis, alleviate wind and resuscitate, relieve spasm to stop pain, eliminate wind and relieve sputum, improve eyesight.

3. 主治 Indications

（1）情志不畅所致的肝气郁结、肝气上逆的病症，如急慢性肝炎、胆囊炎、胆石症、胃脘痛、嗳气、吐酸、上消化道出血等。Acute or chronic hepatitis, cholecystitis, cholelithiasis, epigastralgia, eructation, acid regurgitation, hemorrhage of upper digestive tract, and other diseases or symptoms caused by depression.

（2）各种眼科病症，如急性结膜炎、麦粒肿、视神经萎缩、近视、远视、弱视等。Various ophthalmologic diseases such as acute conjunctivitis, hordeolum, optic atrophy, myopia, hyperopia, amblyopia, etc.

（3）肝血不足或瘀血所致的妇科疾患，如月经不调、痛经、闭经、更年期综合征、脏躁、眩晕、外伤以及血液系统疾病、血管病等。Gynecologic diseases caused by liver-blood deficiency or blood stasis, such as irregular menstruation, dysmenorrhea, amenia, menopausal syndrome, hysteria, dizziness, injury, diseases of blood system, angiopathy, etc.

（4）筋脉拘急、手足抽搐、肢体麻木、关节疼痛等。Spasm of muscles, convulsion of hand and foot, numbness of limbs, arthralgia.

艇中　tingzhong（CO6, 10i）, center of superior concha

1. 定位 Location　在小肠区与肾区之间，即耳甲 6、10 区交界处的中点。Between the point of small intestine and the point of kidney, namely on the juncture between the concha 6 and 10.

2. 功能 Function 理气消胀、消炎止痛。Regulate the circulation of qi, remove flatulence, dephlogisticate, relieve pain.

3. 主治 Indications 腹痛、腹胀、胆道蛔虫症、腮腺炎及水湿不运之症。如：肝硬化腹水、肾炎水肿等。Abdominal pain, abdominal distension, biliary, ascariasis, parotitis, and dysfunction of the circulation of water, such as ascites due to cirrhosis, nephritic edema, etc.

脾　pi（CO13）, spleen

1. 定位 Location 在 BD 线下方，耳甲腔的后上部，即耳甲 13 区。

On the posterior and superior portion of the inferior concha, inferior to the BD line, namely the concha 13.

2. 功能 Function 有运化水谷、健脾补气、统血生肌、清热利湿、补气升提的作用。Be in charge of digestion and transportation, activate the function of the spleen and replenish qi, keep the blood circulating within the blood vessels, clear away dampness and heat, raise splenic qi.

3. 主治 Indications

（1）各种消化系统病症，如消化不良、胃炎、溃疡、小儿厌食 等。Various diseases of alimentary system, such as dyspepsia, gastritis, ulcer, anorexia in children, etc.

（2）脾不健运所致的病症，如营养不良性水肿、慢性肾炎之水肿、功能性水肿、腹水以及痰湿内阻诸证。Diseases caused by spleen dysfunction of removing dampness, such as alimentary edema, chronic nephritic edema, functional edema, ascites, and stagnation of phlegm dampness.

（3）脾不统血所致的各种出血性疾病，如贫血、妇女脾不统血之崩漏、功能性子宫出血。Hemorrhagic syndrome due to dysfunction of keeping the blood within the blood vessels, such as anemia, metrorrhagia and metrostaxis, and functional uterine bleeding.

（4）中气下陷所致的脏器下垂病症，如脱肛、子宫脱垂、慢性腹泻等。Visceroptosis due to abnormal falling of the spleen-qi, proctoptosis, hysteroptosis, chronic diarrhea, etc.

（5）各种原因引起的肌肉萎缩，如进行性脊肌萎缩、进行性肌营养不良症、多发性神经炎恢复期及外伤性失用性肌萎。Various myoatrophy syndrome, progressive spinal myodystrophia, progressive muscle dystrophy, polyneuritis convalescence, and traumatic disabled myoatrophy syndrome.

注：有报道可治梅尼埃病。

Note：It has been reported that this point could be used to treat Meniere's disease.

心　xin（CO15）, heart

1. 定位 Location　在耳甲腔正中凹陷处，即耳甲 15 区。On the central cavity of auricular concha, namely the concha 15.

2. 功能 Function　调节心血管系统及中枢神经系统，具有宁心安神、调和营卫、清泄心火、疏经活络、化瘀止痛、止痒的功能。Regulate the function of cardio vascular system and central nerve system, tranquilize the mind, regulate the function of ying and wei, eliminate heart-fire, activate meridians, clear away blood stasis to stop pain, and relieve itchiness.

3. 主治 Indications

（1）心血管系统病症，如各种心脏病引起的心律紊乱（心动过速、心动过缓、心律不齐等）、心绞痛、无脉症、冠心病、风湿性心脏病。Cardiovascular diseases, such as arrhythmia（tachycardia, bradycardia, arrhythmia）due to various heart diseases, angina pectoris, pulseless disease, coronary heart disease, rheumatic heart disease.

（2）神志异常的病症，如神经官能症、神经衰弱、精神病、癔症、失眠、多梦、健忘、盗汗等。Mental abnormality, such as neurosis, neurasthenia, psychosis, hysteria, insomnia, dreaminess, amnesia, night sweating, etc.

（3）口腔炎、舌炎、慢性咽炎、声音嘶哑等。Stomatitis, glossitis, chronic pharyngitis, hoarseness, etc.

（4）各种疮痒、痛症。Skin and external diseases, pain syndromes.

（5）自汗、多汗、无汗症。Spontaneous perspiration, hyperhidrosis, anhidrosis.

（6）偏瘫、遗精、阳痿、高血压。Hemiparalysis, spermatorrhea, impotence, hypertension.

气管　qiguan（CO16）, trachea

1. 定位 Location　在心区和外耳门之间，即耳甲16区。Between the point of the heart and the point of auditory canal, namely the concha 16.

2. 功能 Function　散风解表、止咳祛痰、止喘利咽。Expel wind and relieve the exterior syndrome, relieve cough and sputum, relieve asthma and sore throat.

3. 主治 Indications　急慢性气管炎、支气管哮喘、喘息样支气管炎、伤风、咳嗽、急性咽炎。Acute or chronic trachitis, bronchial asthma, asthmatic bronchitis, cold, cough and acute pharyngitis.

肺　fei（CO14），lung

1. 定位 Location　在心、气管区周围处，即耳甲 14 区。Peripheral to the portion of the heart and trachea, namely the concha 14.

2. 功能 Function　行气活血、止咳平喘、祛风止痒、利水通便、疏风解表、通鼻开窍。Promote the circulation of qi and blood, relieve cough and asthma, dispel wind and itchiness, promote diuresis and purge, relieve the exterior syndrome, clear away the nasal passage and induce resuscitation.

3. 主治 Indications

（1）呼吸系统病症，如急慢性支气管炎、哮喘、心悸、气短、肺炎、咳嗽、胸闷等。Respiratory diseases, such as acute or chronic bronchitis, bronchial asthma, palpitation, short breath, pneumonia, cough, oppressed feeling in chest, etc.

（2）肺失通调所致的水肿。Edema caused by blocked Lung.

（3）伤风感冒、鼻炎、咽喉炎、盗汗、自汗、脱发、毛发干枯等 Cold, rhinitis, laryngopharyngitis, night sweating, spontaneous perspiration, baldness, tricho-xerosis, etc.

（4）鼻炎、咽炎、声音嘶哑等。Rhinitis, pharyngitis, hoarseness, etc.

（5）过敏性疾病，如急慢性荨麻疹、药物过敏疹、银屑病、带状疱疹、湿疹、痤疮及各种皮肤瘙痒症。Hypersensitive diseases, such as acute or chronic urticaria, drug allergy, psoriasis, herpes zoster, eczema, acne and various cutaneous pruritus, etc.

（6）胃、十二指肠溃疡、便秘、肠炎、泄泻等。
Gastroduodenal ulcer, constipation, enteritis, diarrhea, etc.

注：临床实验表明肺穴有促进溃疡面愈合的作用。

Note：Clinical experiment indicates the point could hasten the heal of the ulcerative surface.

三焦　sanjiao（CO17）, triple energy

1. 定位 Location　在外耳门后下，肺与内分泌区之间，即耳甲17区。Posterior and inferior to the auditory canal, between the point of lung and the point of endocrine, namely the concha 17.

2. 功能 Function　有调节五脏六腑的功能及通利水道的作用，临床上具有流通气血、疏通水道、理气止痛、补心养肺、健脾和胃、补肾利水、滋水止渴的作用。Coordinate the function of five-zang organs and six-fu organs, regulate the fluid passage, activate the circulation of qi and blood, regulate qi to alleviate pain, nourish heart and lung, nourish and regulate spleen and stomach, invigorate kidney to regulate the fluid circulation, nourish water and quench thirst.

3. 主治 Indications

（1）各种内脏器官的病症，如冠心病、胸闷、气短、胁肋疼痛、消化不良、贫血、肝炎等。Various visceral diseases, but such as coronary heart disease, chest distress, short breath, hypochondriac pain, dyspepsia, anemia, hepatitis, etc.

（2）各种原因引起的水肿。Edema due to different reasons.

（3）上肢外侧疼痛。Pain of the lateral side of the upper limbs.

（4）耳鸣、耳聋等。Tinnitus, deafness, etc.

内分泌 neifenmi（CO18）, endocrine

1. 定位 Location　在屏间切迹内，耳甲腔的前下部，即耳甲 18 区。Inside the notch between the tragus and antitragus, on the anterior and inferior portion of the auditory inner concha, namely the concha 18.

2. 功能 Function　有调节内分泌系统各器官的功能，可抗过敏、抗风湿、抗感染、活血通络、调节代谢功能、消肿利湿。Regulate the function of endocrine organs, take effects of anti-anaphylaxis, anti-rheumatic, as well as anti-infection, promote the blood flow, activate the meridians, regulate metabolic function, relieve dampness and subdue swelling.

3. 主治 Indications

（1）内分泌失调引起的各种病症，如甲状腺功能亢进、糖尿病、肥胖症，月经不调、痛经、闭经、更年期综合征，前列腺炎、遗精、不孕不育症。Diseases due to endocrine dysfunction, such as hyperthyrosis, diabetes mellitus, adiposis obesity, irregular menstruation, dysmenorrhea, amenia, menopausal syndrome, prostatitis, spermatorrhea, infertility, etc.

（2）过敏性疾病。如急性荨麻疹、支气管哮喘、药物过敏、湿疹、神经性皮炎、过敏性鼻炎、风湿性关节炎及其他神经炎。Anaphylaxis diseases, such as acute urticaria, bronchial asthma, drug anaphylactic reaction, eczema, neurodermatitis, rhinallergosis rheumatic arthritis, and other neuritis.

（3）吸收代谢功能障碍疾病。如胃炎、消化不良等。Diseases due to dysfunction of digestion and metabolism function, such as gastritis, dyspepsia.

注：对诊断肿瘤有参考意义。

Note：This point is of reference meaning to diagnose tumor.

牙　ya（LO1），tooth

1. 定位 Location　在耳垂正面前上部，即耳垂1区。On the anterior and superior portion of the earlobe grid, namely the earlobe 1.

2. 功能 Function　清热止痛。Clear heat and kill pain.

3. 主治 Indications　牙周炎、低血压。Periodontitis, hypotension.

舌　she（LO2），tongue

1. 定位 Location　在耳垂正面中上部，即耳垂2区。On the middle and superior portion of the earlobe grid, namely the earlobe 2.

2. 功能 Function　清心降火、活血生肌。Clear heat in the heart, promote blood circulation.

3. 主治 Indications　舌炎、舌裂、舌部溃疡、口腔炎等。Glossitis, split tongue, ulcer of tongue, stomatitis.

颌　he（LO3），jaw

1. 定位 Location　在耳垂正面后上部，即耳垂3区。On the posterior and superior portion of the ear lobe grid, namely the earlobe 3.

2. 功能 Function　祛风镇痛。Dispel wind and stop pain.

3. 主治 Indications　各种原因引起的牙痛、颞颌关节炎、颞颌关节功能紊乱、三叉神经痛、牙周炎、牙龈炎、拔牙后反应等。Toothache, temporomandibular arthritis, dysfunction of temporomandibular joint, prosopalgia, periodontitis, gingivitis, postextraction reaction caused by various reasons.

垂前 chuiqian（LO4）, anterior ear lobe

1. 定位 Location 在耳垂正面前中部，即耳垂 4 区。 On the anterior and middle portion of the earlobe grid, namely the earlobe 4.

2. 功能 Function 调节大脑皮层的兴奋和抑制过程，具有镇静安神、止痛的作用。Coordinate the excitement and inhibitation of brain cortex, tranquilize and allay the excitement, arrest pain.

3. 主治 Indications

（1）神经衰弱、头晕、头昏、失眠、多梦、健忘、心悸等。Neurasthenia, dizziness, amnesia, insomnia, dreaminess, palpitation, etc.

（2）牙痛、颞颌关节功能紊乱。Toothache, dysfunction of temporomandibular joint.

注：治疗睡眠时间短，早醒、醒后不易入睡，用此穴疗效佳。

Notes：This point is effective in curing those who suffer poor-quality sleep, wake up early or have difficulty in falling asleep.

眼 yan（LO5）, eye

1. 定位 Location 在耳垂正面中央部，即耳垂 5 区。 On the center of the earlobe grid, namely the ear lobe 5.

2. 功能 Function 清热止痛、疏肝明目。Clear away heat and relieve pain, relieve the depressed liver, smooth the circulation of qi in liver and brighten eyes.

3. 主治 Indications 眼科各种病症，如急性结合膜炎、电光性眼炎、麦粒肿、翼状胬肉、角膜炎、角膜溃疡、虹膜睫状体炎、视网膜炎、视神经萎缩、近视、远视、散光、弱视、青光眼、白内障等。Various ophthalmological diseases, such as acute conjunctivitis, electric ophthalmia, hordeolum, pterygium, keratitis, corneal ulcer, iridocyclitis, retinitis, optic atrophy, myopia, hyperopia, astigmia, amblyopia, glaucoma, cataract, etc.

内耳　neier（LO6），internal ear

1. 定位 Location　在耳垂正面后中部，即耳垂 6 区。On the posterior and middle portion of the earlobe grid, namely the earlobe 6.

2. 功能 Function　祛风清热、通窍聪耳。Dispel wind and heat, improve the function of hearing.

3. 主治 Indications　中耳炎、梅尼埃病及耳鸣、耳聋、听力下降、外耳道疖肿等症。Otitis media, Meniere's disease, deafness, tinnitus, hypoacusis, furuncle of external auditory canal, etc.

面颊　mianjia（LO5.6l），cheek

1. 定位 Location　在耳垂正面眼区与内耳区之间，即耳垂 5、6 区交界处中点。Between the point of eye and the point of internal ear, namely on the juncture between the earlobe 5 and 6.

2. 功能 Function　消炎消肿、祛风止痛、镇痉和改变面部血液循环，是美容要穴。Take effects of anti-inflammation, relieve swelling and pain, dispel wind, relax muscle spasm, improve facial blood circulation, a key point of cosmesis.

3. 主治 Indications　颜面神经麻痹、面神经炎、腮腺炎、三叉神经痛、痤疮、扁平疣、黄褐斑及中老年早衰、面容皱纹增多、面部色素沉着、酒渣鼻。Bell's palsy, facial neuritis, parotitis, prosopalgia, acne, flat wart, chloasma, middle-age senilism, increased facial wrinkles, facial pigmental nevus, brandy nose.

扁桃体　biantaoti（LO7, 8, 9.）, tonsil

1. 定位 Location　在耳垂正面下部，即耳垂 7、8、9 区。On the inferior portion of the earlobe grid, namely the area where the earlobe 7,8,9 are.

2. 功能 Function　清热解毒、消炎、消肿止痛。Clear away heat and toxic substances, take effects of antiinflammation, relieve swelling and pain.

3. 主治 Indications　急慢性扁桃体炎、咽喉炎及各种虚热症。Acute or chronic tonsillitis, pharyngitis, various fevers of deficiency type.

耳背心　erbeixin（P1）, heart of posterior surface

1. 定位 Location　在耳背上部，即耳背 1 区。On the superior portion of the posterior surface of the auricle，namely the posterior earlobe 1.

2. 功能 Function　清泻心火、宁心安神。Clear away the heart-heat, tranquilize the mind.

3. 主治 Indications　心悸、失眠、多梦、高血压、头痛。Palpitation, insomnia, dreaminess, hypertension，headache.

耳背肺　erbeifei（P2）, lung of posterior surface

1. 定位 Location　在耳背中内部，即耳背 2 区。On the middle and internal portion of the posterior surface of the auricle, namely the posterior earlobe 2.

2. 功能 Function　宣肺平喘，止咳，祛风止痒。

Facilitate the flow of lung-qi, relieve asthma, relieve cough, arrest itchiness by dispelling wind.

3. 主治 Indications 气管炎、支气管炎、支气管哮喘、皮肤瘙痒症。Trachitis, bronchitis, bronchial asthma, cutaneous pruritus.

耳背脾 erbeipi（P3）, spleen of posterior surface

1. 定位 Location 在耳背中央部，即耳背3区。On the center of the posterior surface of the auricle, namely the posterior earlobe 3.

2. 功能 Function 健脾和胃、止痛助消化。Improve and regulate the function of the spleen and stomach, relieve pain, improve digestion.

3. 主治 Indications 胃炎、胃及十二指肠溃疡引起的胃痛、消化不良、食欲不振。Gastritis, stomachache due to gastroduodenal ulcer, dyspepsia, poor appetite.

耳背肝 erbeigan（P4）, liver of posterior surface

1. 定位 Location 在耳背中外部，即耳背4区。On the middle and external portion of the auricle, namely the posterior earlobe 4.

2. 功能 Function 疏肝利胆、活络止痛。Relieve depressed liver and gallbladder, promote the circulation of qi, activate meridians to stop pain.

3. 主治 Indications 胆囊炎、胆石症、肝区痛、胁肋痛。Cholecystitis, cholelithiasis, hepatalgia, pain of hypochondriac region.

耳背肾 erbeishen（P5）, kidney of posterior surface

1. 定位 Location 在耳背下部，即耳背5区。On the inferior portion of the posterior surface of the auricle, namely the posterior earlobe 5.

2. 功能 Function 滋补肝肾、强骨益髓、镇静止痛。Nourish liver and kidney, strengthen bone and invigorate marrow, relieve spasm to stop pain.

3. 主治 Indications 各种头痛、头晕、神经衰弱、自主神经功能紊乱、忧郁症、神经官能症。Various headache and dizziness, neurasthenia, dysfunction of autonomic nervous system, melancholy, neurosis.

耳背沟 erbeigou（PS）, groove of posterior surface

1. 定位 Location 在耳背对耳轮沟和对耳轮上、下脚沟处。The groove formed by the antihelix, superior and inferior crus of the antihelix, on the posterior surface of the auricle.

2. 功能 Function 平肝息风、凉血祛风、降压止痒。Calm liver to stop endogenous wind, cool blood to dispel the wind, decrease blood pressure, arrest itchiness.

3. 主治 Indications 高血压、血管性头痛、面神经炎、皮肤瘙痒症。Hypertension, headache, facial neuritis, cutaneous pruritus.

上耳根 shangergen（R1）, upper ear root

1. 定位 Location 在耳根最上处。On the uppermost portion of the ear root.

2. 功能 Function　清热凉血。Clear away blood-heat.

3. 主治 Indications　鼻衄、肌萎缩、各种原因所致瘫痪。Epistaxis, myoatrophy, various paralysis.

耳迷根　ermigen（R2）, root of ear vagus

1. 定位 Location　在耳轮脚后沟起始的耳根处。In the posterior groove formed by the crus of the helix, near the ear root.

2. 功能 Function　清热利湿、通窍止痛、解痉安蛔。Clear away dampness and heat, activate the passage of the five-sense organs and stop pain, relieve spasm and colic caused by ascaris.

3. 主治 Indications　头痛、鼻塞、头晕、失眠、胃痛、腹痛、腹泻、胆石症、落枕、高血压、窦性心动过速、尿潴留、胆道蛔虫症、糖尿病等。Headache, nasal obstruction, insomnia, dizziness, stomachache, abdominal pain, diarrhea, cholelithiasis, hypertension, sinus tachycardia, retention of urine, biliary ascariasis, diabetes mellitus, etc.

下耳根　xiaergen（R3）, lower ear root

1. 定位 Location　在耳根最下处。On the most inferior portion of the ear root.

2. 功能 Function　有提高血压的作用，宁心安神，滋补肝肾。Increase the blood pressure, tranquilize the mind, relieve mental stress, nourish liver and kidney.

3. 主治 Indications　低血压、内分泌功能紊乱、面瘫、面痛。Hypotension, endocrine disturbance, Bell's palsy, prosopodynia.

经验耳穴

The Empirical Auricular Points

便秘点　bianmidian, constipation point

1. 定位 Location　三角窝中 1/3，对耳轮下脚中段的上缘坐骨神经点的上方。On the middle one-third of the triangular fossa, along the superior edge of the middle part of the inferior crus of the antihelix, superior to the point of the sciatic nerve.

2. 功能 Function　可促进大肠的蠕动。Promote the laxation of the large intestine.

3. 主治 Indications　痔疮、便秘、便血。Hemorrhoid, constipation, hematochezia.

胰腺炎点　yixianyandian, pancreatitis point

1. 定位 Location　在十二指肠穴与胰胆穴两穴连线的中下 1/3 交界处。On the middle and inferior one-third of the juncture between the point of duodenum and the point of pancreas and gallbladder.

2. 功能 Function　解痛消炎、通络止痛。Take effects of antiinflammation, activate the meridians, arrest pain.

3. 主治 Indications　急慢性胰腺炎、消化不良、上腹胀满、糖尿病。Acute and chronic pancreatitis, dyspepsia, epigastric distention, diabetes.

兴奋点　xingfendian, excitation point

1. 定位 Location　在对耳屏内侧面与耳甲腔交界处。On the juncture between the superior concha and internal side of the antitragus.

2. 功能 Function　增强大脑皮层的兴奋过程。Enhance the excitement of the cortex.

3. 主治 Indications　嗜睡以及由此引起的遗尿、精神萎靡、内分泌及性功能低下、闭经、阳痿以及肥胖症等。Lethargy, and enuresis, restlessness, endocrine system hypofunction, sexual hypofunction, amenia, impotence, obesity caused by lethargy.

渴点　kedian, thirst point

1. 定位 Location　在屏尖与外鼻两穴的中点偏上处。Slightly superior to the midpoint between the apex of the tragus and the point of the external nose.

2. 功能 Function　有清泻三焦之火、泄脾热胃火、滋肾壮水的作用（抑制摄水）。Remove the upper-jiao heat, relieve the gastric heat, nourish kidney to strengthen the renal yin（inhibit the intake of water）.

3. 主治 Indications　尿崩症、糖尿病及其他原因引起的消渴、烦渴等症，还可用于神经性多饮及肥胖症。Polydipsia or excessive thirst caused by diabetes insipidus, diabetes mellitus and other diseases, may also be applied to treat nervous polydipsia and obesity.

饥点　jidian, hunger point

1. 定位 Location　在肾上腺与外鼻两穴的中点偏下处。Slightly inferior to the midpoint between the point of adrenal gland and the point of external nose.

2. 功能 Function　有控制饮食、抗风湿、抗过敏的作用。Control diet，anti-rheumatism, antianaphylaxis, relieve gastric heat.

3. 主治 Indications　胃热亢盛所致的消谷善饥之症，泄泻、全身无力，并对胃肠功能紊乱、过敏性结肠炎有一定疗效，还可治疗肥胖症及甲状腺功能亢进、糖尿病等。
Bulimia induced by stomach-heat, diarrhea, fatigue, some effects on gastrointestinal disorder, allergic colitis, as well as obesity and hyperthyrosis, diabetes, etc.

卵巢　luanchao, ovary

1. 定位 Location　在对耳屏皮质下穴的前下方。Anterior and inferior to the point of the subcortex, on the antitragus.

2. 功能 Function　有滋阴补肾、调节卵巢功能的作用。Nourish kidney and liver, regulate ovarian function.

3. 主治 Indications　卵巢及子宫疾患。如月经不调、痛经、附件炎、卵巢炎、输卵管炎、不孕症、性功能障碍、阳痿、肾虚性腰痛、功能性子宫出血。Ovarian and uterine diseases, such as irregular menstruation, dysmenorrhea, adnexitis, ovaritis, salpingitis, acyesis, hypogonadism, impotence, lumbago due to deficiency of kidney, functional uterine bleeding, etc.

乳腺　ruxian, breast

1. 定位 Location　耳轮脚消失处延线与胸穴相交处。两个并列的穴点。On the junction of crus of helix vanishing extension and chest point.

2. 功能 Function　活血消炎，通乳止痛。Promote blood flow, diminish inflammation, promoting lactation, stop pain.

3. 主治 Indications　乳腺增生、急慢性乳腺炎、乳痈、乳汁少、乳汁排出不畅等乳腺疾病。Hyperplasia of the mammary glands, acute and chronic mastitis, lack of lactation, lactation disturbance, etc.

睾丸 gaowan, testis

1. 定位 Location 在对耳屏、皮质下穴的后下方。Posterior and inferior to the point of the subcortex, on the antitragus.

2. 功能 Function 益肾壮阳、消肿止痛。Nourish kidney and strengthen renal yang, alleviate edema and stop pain.

3. 主治 Indications 生殖系统病症。如睾丸炎、神经衰弱、性功能障碍、阴囊湿疹、再生障碍性贫血、前列腺炎、不孕症等。Reproductive system diseases, such as orchitis, neurasthenia, sexual disorder, eczema of scrotum, aplastic anemia, prostatitis, acyesis, etc.

枕小神经 zhenxiaoshenjing, nervus occipitalis minor

1. 定位 Location 位于耳轮结节上缘约 0.2cm 之内侧面。On the interior surface of the auricle, 0.2cm superior to the helix tubercle.

2. 功能 Function 有镇静止痛、通经活络和调节脑血管运动的作用。Alleviate pain，activate the meridians，regulate the function of cerebrovascular movement.

3. 主治 Indications 头痛、枕大神经痛、耳廓痛、脑血管痉挛、脑外伤后遗症、脑动脉硬化、神经官能症引起的半身麻木及头部麻木等。Headache, greater occipital nerve pain, auricular neuralgia, cerebrovascular spasm, sequel of cerebral injury, cerebral arteriosclerosis, hemianesthesia, etc.

甲状腺 1 jiazhuangxian1, thyroid 1

1. 定位 Location 在颈椎穴的外上方，与颈穴平。Exterior and superior to the point of cervical vertebrae, paralleled to the point of neck.

2. 功能 Function　可调节甲状腺功能、升高血压、增强大脑皮层的抑制程度。Regulate thyroid function, elevate blood pressure, enhance inhibition of cerebral cortex.

3. 主治 Indications　甲状腺疾患，如甲状腺瘤、甲状腺功能亢进，甲状腺功能减退，低血压、神经衰弱等。Thyroid diseases, such as thyrophyma, hyperthyrosis, hypothyrosis, hypotension, neurasthenia, etc.

甲状腺2　jiazhuangxian2, thyroid 2

1. 定位 Location　内耳穴内上方靠近面颊区处。On the inside of the above of internal ear point, clear to the cheek point.

2. 功能 Function　调节甲状腺功能、升高血压、增强大脑皮层的抑制程度。Regulate thyroid function ,elevate blood pressure, enhance inhibition of cerebral cortex.

3. 主治 Indications　甲状腺疾病，如甲状腺瘤，甲状腺功能亢进或减退，神经衰弱，低血压等。Thyroid diseases, such as thyrophyma, hyperthyrosis, hypothyroidism, neurasthenia, hypotension, etc.

心脏点　xinzangdian, viscera point

1. 定位 Location　在屏尖穴与外耳穴连线的中点。The midpoint between the point of tragus apex and the external ear.

2. 功能 Function　是降心率的经验穴，有调节心律的作用。Empirical point of decreasing heart rate, regulate heart rhythm.

3. 主治 Indications　心律失常、阵发性心动过速、房颤。Arrhythmia, paroxysmal tachycardia, atrial fibrillation.

注：临床观察对心动过缓也有一定的疗效。

Note：Clinical experiment indicates that the point could be effective in treating bradycardia.

肾炎点　shenyandian, nephritis point

1. 定位 Location　耳舟下部，锁骨穴外下方，偏耳轮处。On the inferior portion of the scaphoid fossa, external and inferior to the point of clavicle, near the helix.

2. 功能 Function　消炎、利水、止痛。Antiinflammation, alleviate water retention, stop pain.

3. 主治 Indications　肾盂肾炎、肾小球肾炎等肾脏疾患。Diseases of kidney, such as pyelitis, glomerulonephritis, etc.

注：是诊断肾小球肾炎的主要参考穴。

Note：It's an important reference point to diagnose glomerulonephritis.

失眠穴　shimianxue, insomnia point

1. 定位 Location　在耳轮脚后沟尾部与对耳轮后沟交界处。On the juncture between the rear of the posterior groove of the crus and the antihelix.

2. 功能 Function　有较强的镇静、安神作用。Tranquilize and allay excitement.

3. 主治 Indications　失眠（入睡慢）Insomnia（having difficulty falling asleep）。

注：当用耳廓正面穴位治疗失眠效果不佳时，改用此穴常获奇效。

Note：It might be especially effective in insomnia treatment when the points on frontal auricle are not working.

高血压点 gaoxueyadian, hypertension point

1. 定位 Location 在肾上腺与屏间前穴两穴的中点偏前方。On the anterior to the midpoint of the juncture between the point of adrenal gland and the point of anterior intertragal notch.

2. 功能 Function 镇静、安神、降血压。Tranquilize and allay excitement, lower the blood pressure.

3. 主治 Indications 高血压，也可治冠心病、头昏头晕、头痛。Hypertension, as well as coronary heart disease, dizziness, headache.

热穴 rexue, heat point

1. 定位 Location 位于腰骶椎穴的上 2/5 与下 3/5 交界线的中点。On the midpoint of the juncture between superior two-fifths and three-fifths of the portion of the lumbosacral vertebrae.

2. 功能 Function 有镇痛、退热和扩张血管的作用。Relieve pain, clear away the heat, and expand the vessel.

3. 主治 Indications 阳虚血脉失于温运的病症。能改善末梢血液循环，提高皮肤温度。常用于治疗无脉症、血栓闭塞性脉管炎、静脉炎、雷诺病、急性腰扭伤等。Diseases and symptoms caused by deficiency of yang and shortage of warm in the meridians. Improve the peripheral circulation and the skin temperature. Usually used to treat pulseless disease, thromboangitis obliterans, phlebitis, Raynaud diseases, acute lumbar sprain, ect.

低血压点 dixueyadian, hypotension point

1. 定位 Location 屏间切迹正中稍下方。Slightly interior to the midpoint of the notch between the tragus and antitragus.

2. 功能 Function 升血压。Increase the blood pressure.

3. 主治 Indications 低血压，尤以对因硬脊膜外麻醉引起的血压降低有较理想的治疗作用。Hypotension, especially used for low blood pressure due to epidural block anesthesia.

新眼 1 xinyan1, new eye 1

定位 Location 屏间切迹正中线向内向后 0.2cm。0.2cm anterior and interior to the notch between the tragus and antitragus.

新眼 2 xinyan2, new eye 2

定位 Location 食道穴和贲门穴连线中点向下和肺区交界处。On the juncture between the point of lung and the midpoint between the point of esophagus and the point of cardia.

新眼 3 xinyan3, new eye 3

定位 Location 在三角窝中 1/3 靠近后 1/3 边缘处。On the middle one-third of the triangular fossa, near the edge of the posterior one-third.

新眼 4 xinyan4, new eye 4

定位 Location 耳轮结节穴的内侧面。On the interior

side of the point of tubercle.

明亮　mingliang, bright

定位 Location　在耳背后相当于耳背肝处"<"字形的凹陷中。In the "<" shaped groove, on the posterior surface of the auricle, where is also the point of the liver in the posterior surface.

后眼 1　houyan1, eye of back auricle 1

定位 Location　在耳背后下有"V"字形的凹陷中。In the "v" shaped groove on the posterior surface of the auricle.

后眼　houyan, eye of back auricle

定位 Location　耳垂正面眼穴的耳垂背面。On the back of the earlobe grid, level with the point of eye.

注：以上 6 穴系编者治疗眼科疾病的经验穴，有滋补肝肾、调节气血平衡、益气明目的作用。

Notes：All the six points mentioned above are empirical points established from our long-term clinical practice. They could be applied to treat ophthalmic diseases, functioning to nourish liver and kidney, coordinate the balance between qi and blood, benefit qi and enhance eyesight.

常见疾病耳穴处方应用图卡

The Auricular Point Formula Memory
Card for Common Diseases

阵发性心动过速
Paroxysmal Tachycardia

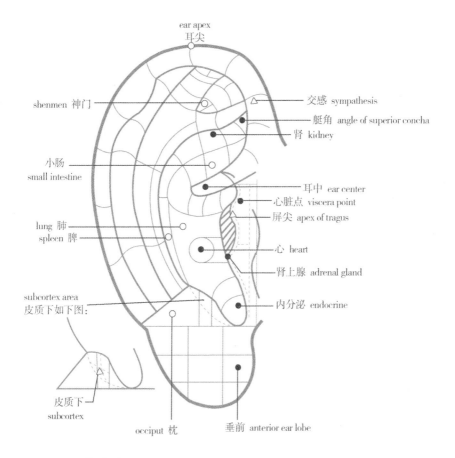

ear apex 耳尖

shenmen 神门

交感 sympathesis

艇角 angle of superior concha

肾 kidney

小肠 small intestine

耳中 ear center

心脏点 viscera point

屏尖 apex of tragus

lung 肺 spleen 脾

心 heart

肾上腺 adrenal gland

subcortex area 皮质下如下图:

内分泌 endocrine

皮质下 subcortex

occiput 枕

垂前 anterior ear lobe

●主穴

心、心脏点、耳中、肾、内分泌、垂前、艇角、肾上腺

○配穴

交感、神门、皮质下、耳尖、小肠、枕、脾、肺、屏尖

房颤
Atrial Fibrillation

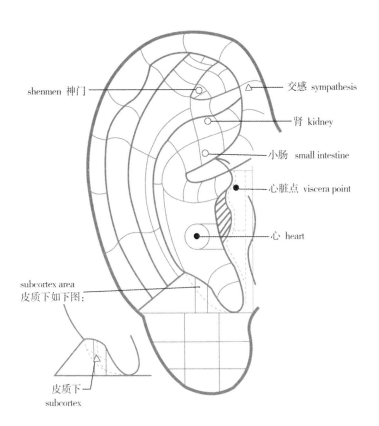

shenmen 神门
交感 sympathesis
肾 kidney
小肠 small intestine
心脏点 viscera point
心 heart
subcortex area
皮质下如下图：
皮质下
subcortex

●主穴

心、心脏点

○配穴

神门、小肠、交感、皮质下、肾

高血压
Hypertension

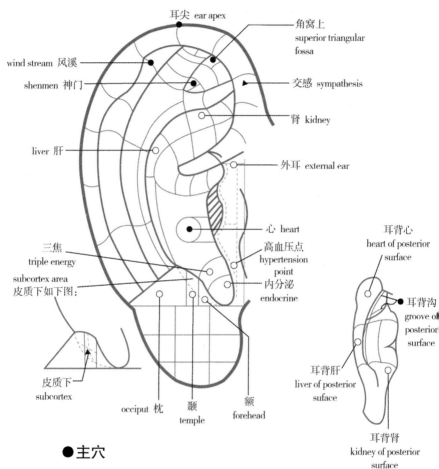

●主穴

角窝上、耳背沟、心、神门、耳尖、皮质下、交感、风溪

○配穴

内分泌、颞、额、肝、肾、高血压点、外耳、枕、三焦、耳背心、耳背肝、耳背肾

低血压
Hypotension

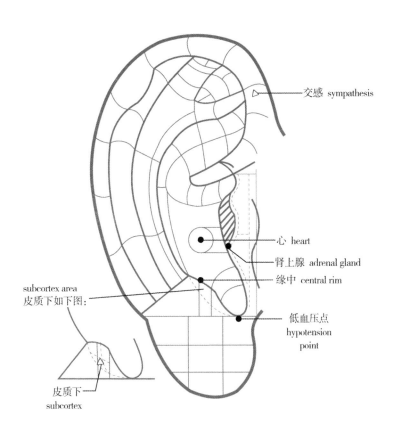

交感 sympathesis

心 heart

肾上腺 adrenal gland

缘中 central rim

低血压点
hypotension
point

subcortex area
皮质下如下图:

皮质下
subcortex

●主穴

肾上腺、低血压点、缘中、心

○配穴

皮质下、交感

风湿性心脏病
Rheumatic Heart Disease

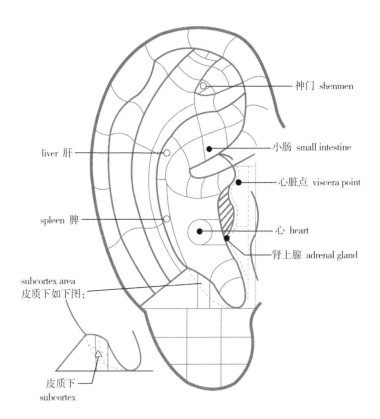

神门 shenmen

小肠 small intestine

心脏点 viscera point

liver 肝

心 heart

肾上腺 adrenal gland

spleen 脾

subcortex area
皮质下如下图:

皮质下
subcortex

● **主穴**

心、小肠、肾上腺、心脏点

○ **配穴**

皮质下、神门、脾、肝

冠心病
Coronary Heart Disease

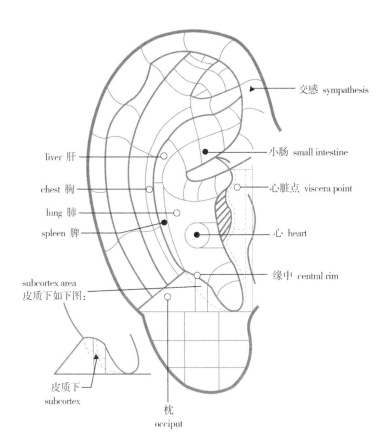

交感 sympathesis

小肠 small intestine

liver 肝

chest 胸

lung 肺

spleen 脾

心脏点 viscera point

心 heart

subcortex area
皮质下如下图:

缘中 central rim

皮质下
subcortex

枕
occiput

●主穴

心、小肠、交感、皮质下、脾

○配穴

缘中、肺、胸、心脏点、枕、肝

无脉症
Pulseless Disease

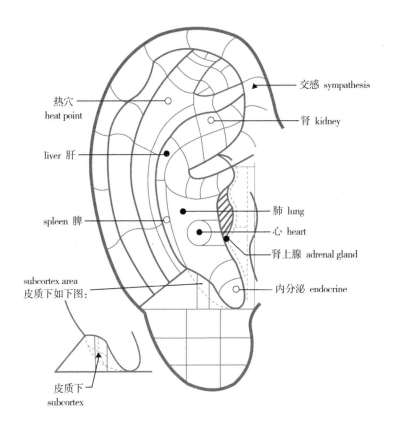

热穴 heat point

交感 sympathesis

肾 kidney

liver 肝

spleen 脾

肺 lung

心 heart

肾上腺 adrenal gland

subcortex area
皮质下如下图：

内分泌 endocrine

皮质下
subcortex

●**主穴**

心、交感、肝、肾上腺、肺、皮质下

○**配穴**

内分泌、脾、肾、热穴

心肌炎
Myocarditis

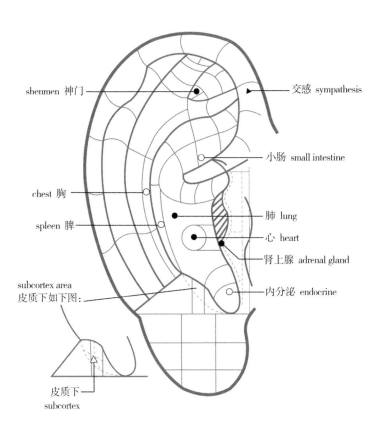

shenmen 神门 —
chest 胸 —
spleen 脾 —
subcortex area 皮质下如下图:—
皮质下
subcortex

交感 sympathesis
小肠 small intestine
肺 lung
心 heart
肾上腺 adrenal gland
内分泌 endocrine

●主穴

心、交感、肾上腺、神门、肺

○配穴

脾、小肠、胸、皮质下、内分泌

心动过缓
Bradycardia

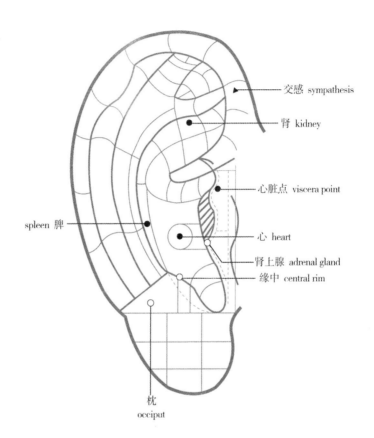

交感 sympathesis

肾 kidney

心脏点 viscera point

spleen 脾

心 heart

肾上腺 adrenal gland

缘中 central rim

枕
occiput

●主穴

心、心脏点、肾、交感、脾

○配穴

枕、缘中、肾上腺

血小板减少性紫癜
Thrombocytopenic Purpura

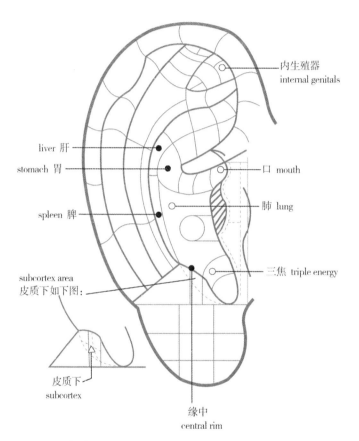

内生殖器
internal genitals

liver 肝

stomach 胃

口 mouth

spleen 脾

肺 lung

subcortex area
皮质下如下图：

三焦 triple energy

皮质下
subcortex

缘中
central rim

●主穴

肝、脾、胃、缘中

○配穴

口、皮质下、三焦、肺、内生殖器

白细胞减少症
Leucocytopenia

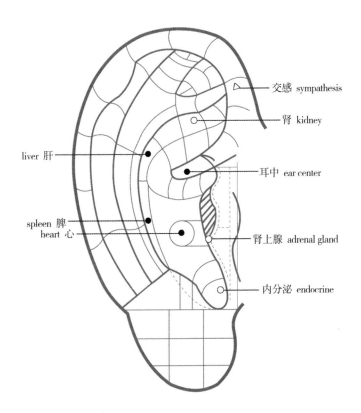

交感 sympathesis

肾 kidney

liver 肝

耳中 ear center

spleen 脾
heart 心

肾上腺 adrenal gland

内分泌 endocrine

●主穴

心、肝、脾、耳中

○配穴

内分泌、肾、肾上腺、交感

肺结核
Pulmonary Tuberculosis

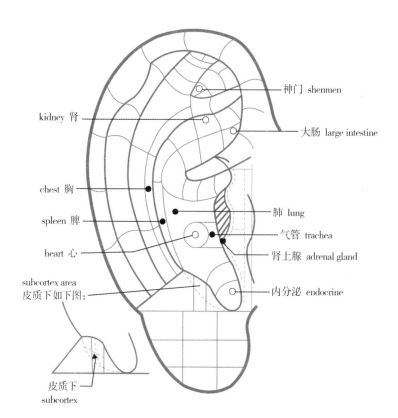

●主穴

肺、气管、脾、肾上腺、胸、皮质下

○配穴

肾、心、内分泌、神门、大肠

支气管哮喘
Bronchial Asthma

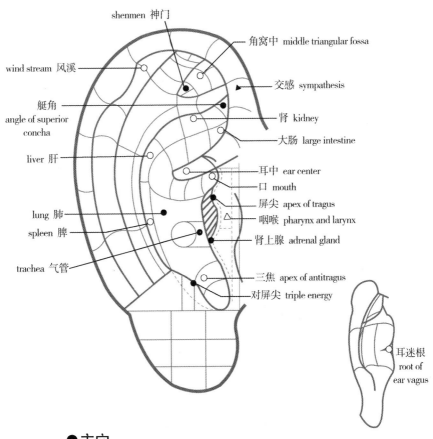

shenmen 神门

角窝中 middle triangular fossa

wind stream 风溪

交感 sympathesis

艇角
angle of superior concha

肾 kidney

大肠 large intestine

liver 肝

耳中 ear center

口 mouth

屏尖 apex of tragus

lung 肺

咽喉 pharynx and larynx

spleen 脾

肾上腺 adrenal gland

trachea 气管

三焦 apex of antitragus

对屏尖 triple energy

耳迷根
root of ear vagus

●主穴

肺、气管、肾上腺、对屏尖、神门、交感、艇角、屏尖

○配穴

脾、肾、三焦、大肠、咽喉、肝、耳迷根、风溪、口、角窝中、耳中

急性支气管炎
Acute Bronchitis

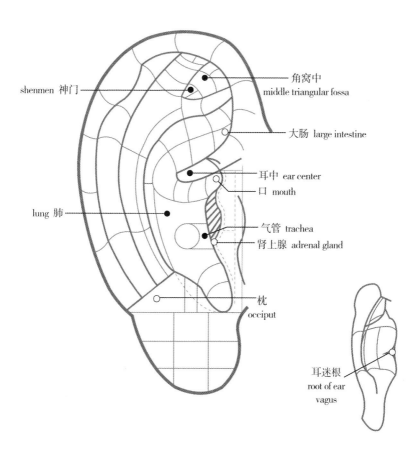

shenmen 神门

角窝中 middle triangular fossa

大肠 large intestine

耳中 ear center
口 mouth

lung 肺

气管 trachea
肾上腺 adrenal gland

枕 occiput

耳迷根 root of ear vagus

●主穴

肺、气管、神门、角窝中、耳中

○配穴

枕、肾上腺、耳迷根、大肠、口

慢性支气管炎
Chronic Bronchitis

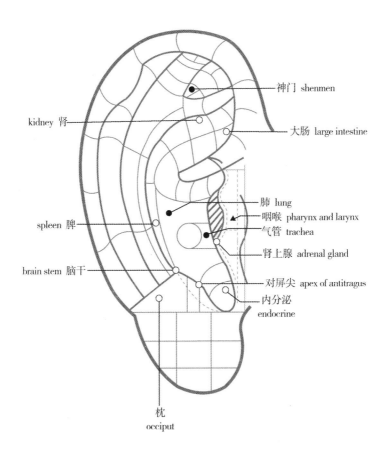

神门 shenmen

kidney 肾

大肠 large intestine

肺 lung
咽喉 pharynx and larynx
气管 trachea

spleen 脾

肾上腺 adrenal gland

brain stem 脑干

对屏尖 apex of antitragus
内分泌
endocrine

枕
occiput

●主穴

肺、神门、气管、咽喉

○配穴

对屏尖、大肠、脾、肾、内分泌、脑干、枕、肾上腺

咳嗽
Cough

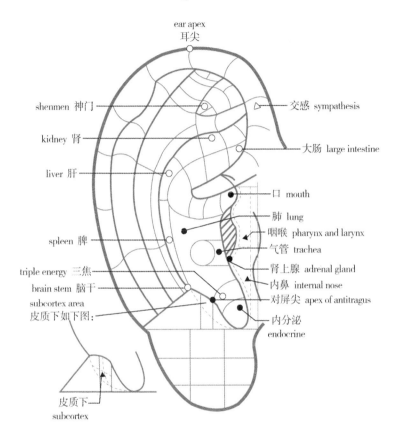

●**主穴**

气管、咽喉、口、对屏尖、肺、肾上腺、内鼻、内分泌

○**配穴**

神门、脾、大肠、肾、交感、脑干、皮质下、肝、耳尖、三焦

咳血
Hemoptysis

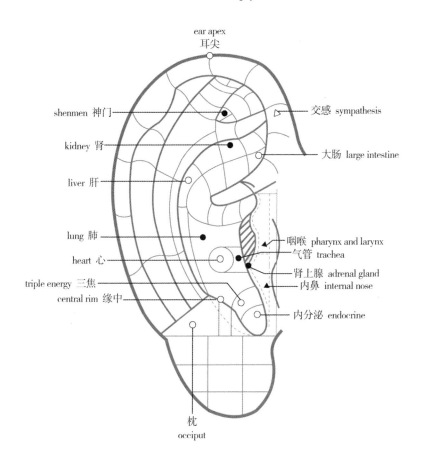

ear apex
耳尖

shenmen 神门

交感 sympathesis

kidney 肾

大肠 large intestine

liver 肝

lung 肺

咽喉 pharynx and larynx
气管 trachea

heart 心

肾上腺 adrenal gland
内鼻 internal nose

triple energy 三焦

central rim 缘中

内分泌 endocrine

枕
occiput

●主穴

气管、肺、神门、咽喉、内鼻、肾上腺、肾

○配穴

交感、三焦、枕、大肠、肝、内分泌、耳尖、缘中、心

急、慢性肝炎
Acute and Chronic Hepatitis

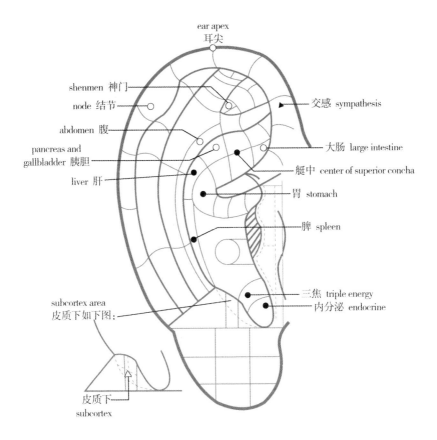

●主穴

肝、脾、胃、艇中、三焦、交感、内分泌

○配穴

胰胆、神门、皮质下、大肠、腹、结节、耳尖

呃逆
Hiccup

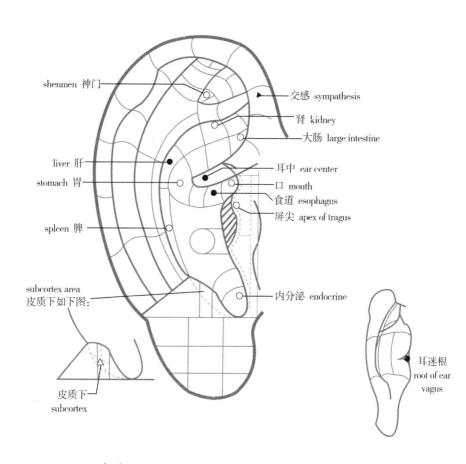

shenmen 神门
交感 sympathesis
肾 kidney
大肠 large intestine
liver 肝
耳中 ear center
stomach 胃
口 mouth
食道 esophagus
屏尖 apex of tragus
spleen 脾
subcortex area
皮质下如下图:
内分泌 endocrine
皮质下
subcortex
耳迷根
root of ear
vagus

●主穴

耳中、耳迷根、交感、食道、肝

○配穴

胃、口、神门、皮质下、肾、内分泌、屏尖、脾、大肠

恶心、呕吐
Nausea and Vomiting

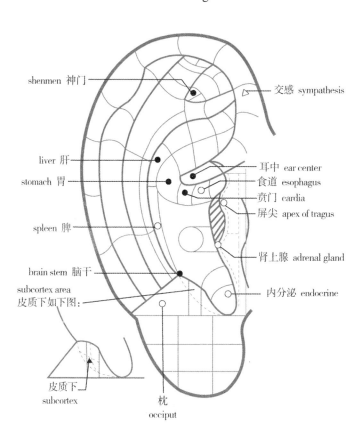

shenmen 神门

交感 sympathesis

liver 肝

耳中 ear center
食道 esophagus
贲门 cardia
屏尖 apex of tragus

stomach 胃

spleen 脾

肾上腺 adrenal gland

brain stem 脑干

subcortex area
皮质下如下图：

内分泌 endocrine

皮质下
subcortex

枕
occiput

● **主穴**

胃、肝、脾、神门、耳中、皮质下、贲门

○ **配穴**

枕、交感、食道、脑干、肾上腺、屏尖、内分泌

便秘
Constipation

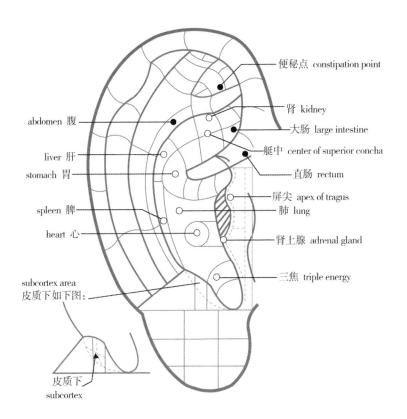

便秘点 constipation point

肾 kidney

abdomen 腹

大肠 large intestine

艇中 center of superior concha

liver 肝

stomach 胃

直肠 rectum

spleen 脾

屏尖 apex of tragus

肺 lung

heart 心

肾上腺 adrenal gland

三焦 triple energy

subcortex area
皮质下如下图:

皮质下
subcortex

●主穴

大肠、直肠、便秘点、皮质下、腹

○配穴

三焦、肾、脾、肺、胃、艇中、肝、心、屏尖、肾上腺

急性腹泻
Acute Diarrhea

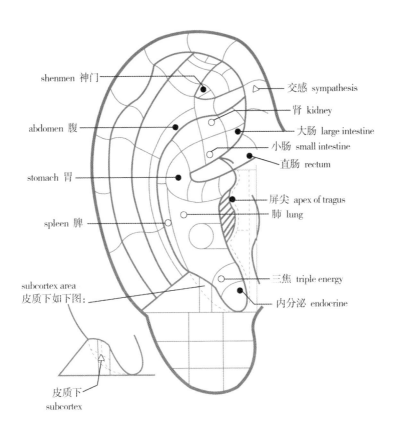

shenmen 神门

abdomen 腹

stomach 胃

spleen 脾

subcortex area
皮质下如下图：

皮质下
subcortex

交感 sympathesis

肾 kidney

大肠 large intestine

小肠 small intestine

直肠 rectum

屏尖 apex of tragus

肺 lung

三焦 triple energy

内分泌 endocrine

●主穴

胃、大肠、直肠、腹、内分泌、神门、屏尖

○配穴

脾、小肠、交感、皮质下、肺、肾、三焦

急、慢性胃炎
Chronic and Acute Gastritis

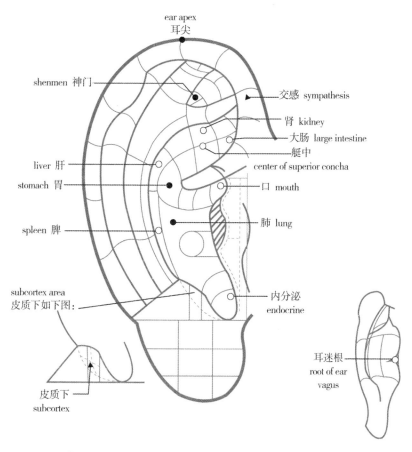

●主穴

胃、交感、肺、皮质下、神门、耳尖

○配穴

肝、脾、口、内分泌、耳迷根、艇中、大肠、肾

胃、十二指肠溃疡
Gastric and Duodenal ulcer

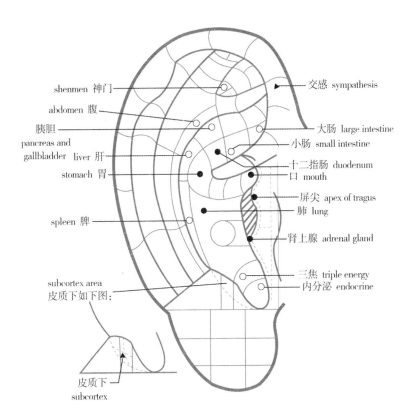

shenmen 神门
abdomen 腹
胰胆
pancreas and
gallbladder liver 肝
stomach 胃
spleen 脾
subcortex area
皮质下如下图：
皮质下
subcortex

交感 sympathesis
大肠 large intestine
小肠 small intestine
十二指肠 duodenum
口 mouth
屏尖 apex of tragus
肺 lung
肾上腺 adrenal gland
三焦 triple energy
内分泌 endocrine

●主穴

胃、十二指肠、交感、皮质下、肺、口、肾上腺、屏尖

○配穴

三焦、神门、腹、肝、大肠、脾、胰胆、内分泌、小肠

溃疡性结肠炎
Ulcerative Colitis

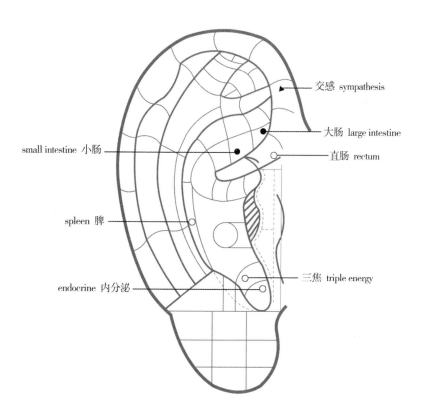

交感 sympathesis

大肠 large intestine

small intestine 小肠

直肠 rectum

spleen 脾

endocrine 内分泌

三焦 triple energy

● 主穴

大肠、小肠、交感

○ 配穴

脾、直肠、三焦、内分泌

胃神经官能症
Gastrointestinal Neurosis

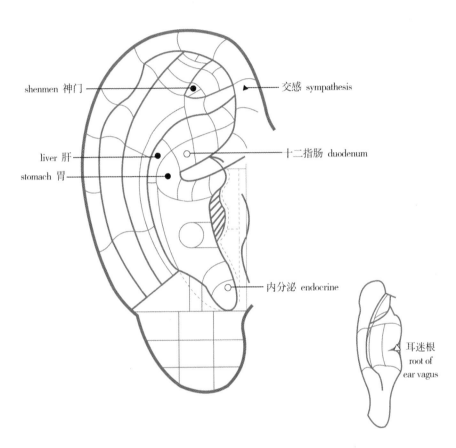

shenmen 神门
交感 sympathesis
liver 肝
十二指肠 duodenum
stomach 胃
内分泌 endocrine
耳迷根 root of ear vagus

●主穴

胃、神门、交感、肝

○配穴

内分泌、十二指肠、耳迷根

胃痉挛
Gastrospasm

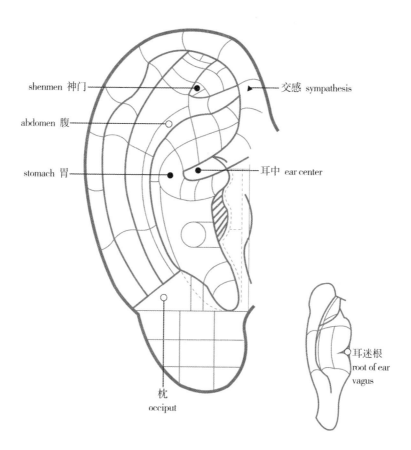

shenmen 神门

abdomen 腹

stomach 胃

交感 sympathesis

耳中 ear center

枕
occiput

耳迷根
root of ear
vagus

● 主穴

胃、神门、交感、耳中

○ 配穴

腹、枕、耳迷根

慢性胆囊炎
Chronic Cholecystitis

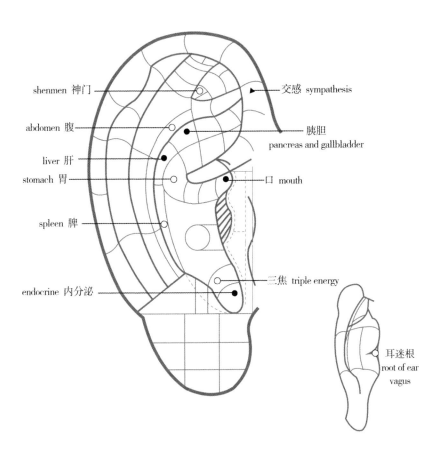

shenmen 神门

abdomen 腹

liver 肝

stomach 胃

spleen 脾

endocrine 内分泌

交感 sympathesis

胰胆
pancreas and gallbladder

口 mouth

三焦 triple energy

耳迷根
root of ear
vagus

●主穴

胰胆、肝、交感、内分泌

○配穴

神门、耳迷根、口、脾、三焦、胃、腹

胆石症
Cholelithiasis

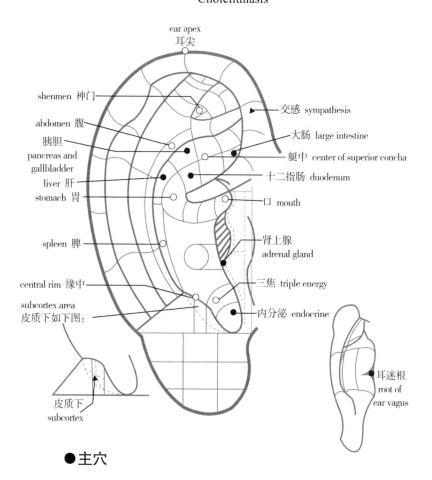

●主穴

　　肝、胰胆、十二指肠、肾上腺、交感、内分泌、大肠、
耳迷根

○配穴

　　神门、腹、胃、口、艇中、皮质下、缘中、三焦、耳尖、脾

慢性胰腺炎
Chronic Pancreatitis

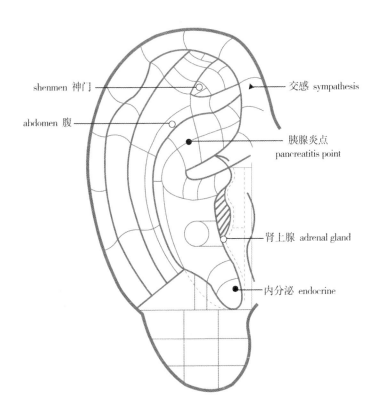

shenmen 神门

abdomen 腹

交感 sympathesis

胰腺炎点
pancreatitis point

肾上腺 adrenal gland

内分泌 endocrine

●主穴

胰腺炎点、内分泌、交感

○配穴

神门、肾上腺、腹

胃肠功能失调
Gastrointestinal Dysfunction

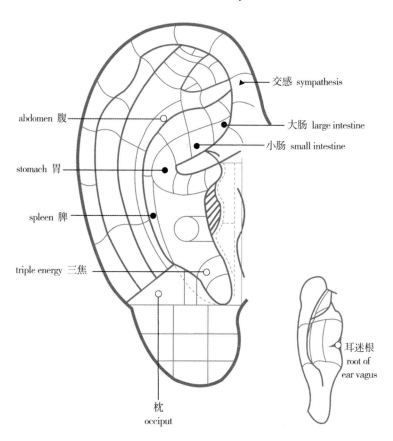

abdomen 腹

stomach 胃

spleen 脾

triple energy 三焦

交感 sympathesis

大肠 large intestine

小肠 small intestine

耳迷根
root of
ear vagus

枕
occiput

●主穴

胃、交感、脾、大肠、小肠

○配穴

腹、三焦、耳迷根、枕

细菌性痢疾
Bacillary Dysentery

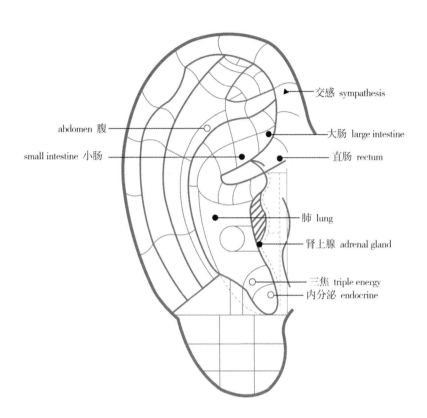

●主穴

大肠、小肠、肺、直肠、交感、肾上腺

○配穴

三焦、内分泌、腹

阑尾炎
Appendicitis

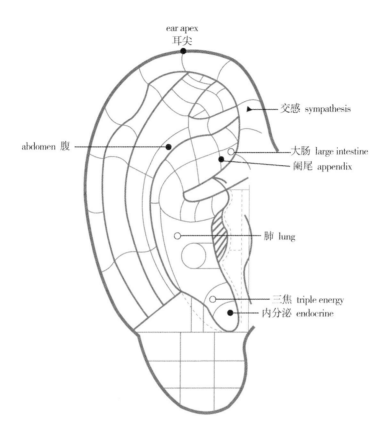

●**主穴**

阑尾、腹、交感、内分泌、耳尖

○**配穴**

肺、大肠、三焦

胆道蛔虫症
Biliary Ascariasis

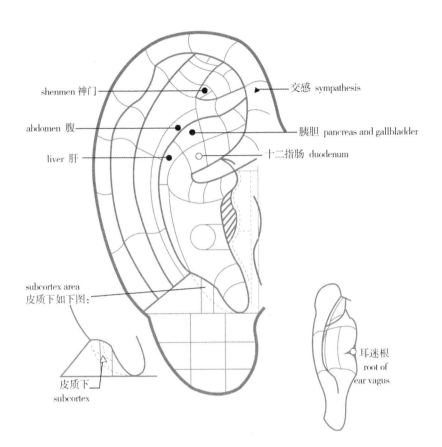

shenmen 神门

交感 sympathesis

abdomen 腹

胰胆 pancreas and gallbladder

liver 肝

十二指肠 duodenum

subcortex area
皮质下如下图：

皮质下
subcortex

耳迷根
root of
ear vagus

●主穴

胰胆、交感、神门、肝、腹

○配穴

十二指肠、耳迷根、皮质下

小儿积滞
Infantile Malnutrition

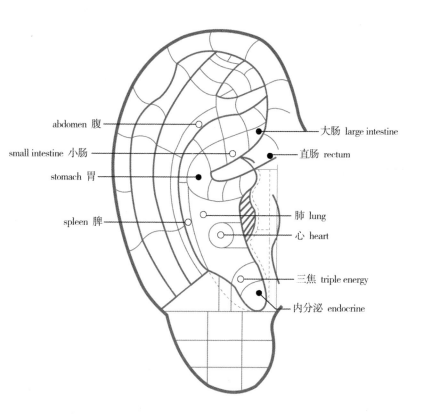

abdomen 腹

small intestine 小肠

stomach 胃

spleen 脾

大肠 large intestine

直肠 rectum

肺 lung

心 heart

三焦 triple energy

内分泌 endocrine

●主穴

胃、大肠、直肠、内分泌

○配穴

心、肺、三焦、脾、小肠、腹

小儿厌食
Infantile Anorexia

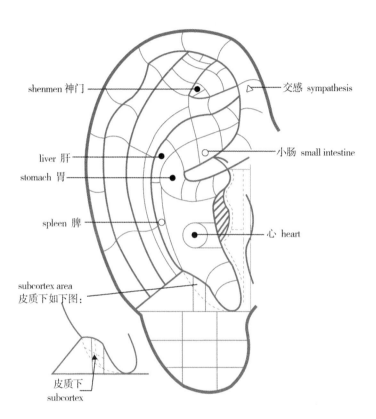

shenmen 神门
交感 sympathesis
liver 肝
小肠 small intestine
stomach 胃
spleen 脾
心 heart
subcortex area
皮质下如下图：
皮质下
subcortex

●主穴

胃、神门、皮质下、肝、心

○配穴

脾、小肠、交感

胃下垂
Gastroptosis

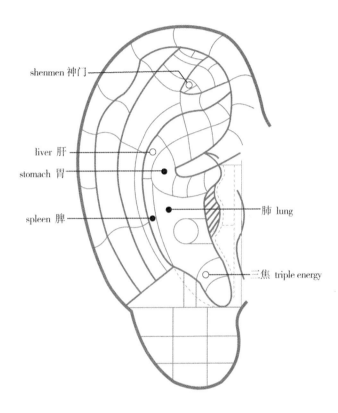

shenmen 神门

liver 肝
stomach 胃

spleen 脾

肺 lung

三焦 triple energy

●主穴

胃、脾、肺

○配穴

三焦、神门、肝

头痛
Headache

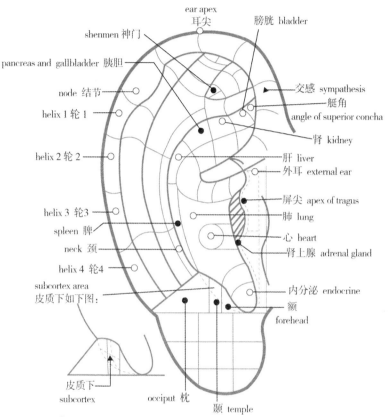

●主穴

额、颞、枕、神门、皮质下、胰胆、交感、肾上腺、屏尖、脾

○配穴

颈、心、肝、耳尖、轮 1 ~ 轮 4、肾、外耳、膀胱、肺、内分泌、结节、艇角

神经衰弱
Neurosism

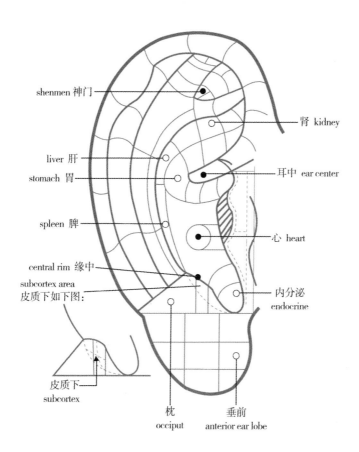

shenmen 神门

肾 kidney

liver 肝
stomach 胃

耳中 ear center

spleen 脾

心 heart

central rim 缘中
subcortex area
皮质下如下图:

内分泌
endocrine

皮质下
subcortex

枕
occiput

垂前
anterior ear lobe

●主穴

心、神门、皮质下、缘中、耳中

○配穴

肾、脾、肝、内分泌、胃、垂前、枕

癔症
Hysteria

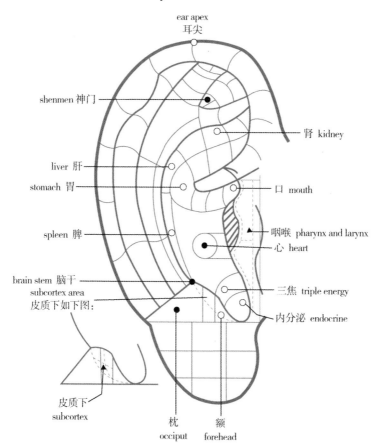

●主穴

心、皮质下、枕、脑干、神门、咽喉

○配穴

肝、内分泌、额、口、脾、胃、三焦、耳尖、肾

失眠
Insomnia

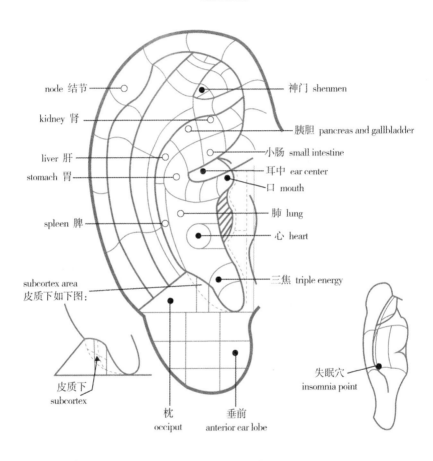

node 结节
kidney 肾
liver 肝
stomach 胃
spleen 脾
subcortex area
皮质下如下图:
皮质下
subcortex

神门 shenmen
胰胆 pancreas and gallbladder
小肠 small intestine
耳中 ear center
口 mouth
肺 lung
心 heart
三焦 triple energy

失眠穴
insomnia point

枕
occiput

垂前
anterior ear lobe

●主穴

心、神门、枕、皮质下、口、失眠穴、三焦、垂前、耳中

○配穴

肝、脾、结节、胃、胰胆、肾、肺、小肠

内分泌失调
Endocrine Dysfunction

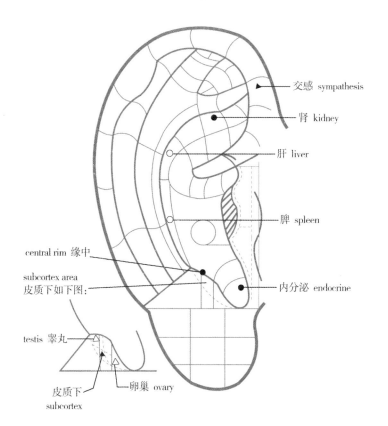

●主穴

内分泌、缘中、皮质下、肾、交感

○配穴

肝、脾、睾丸（男）、卵巢（女）

癫痫
Epilepsy

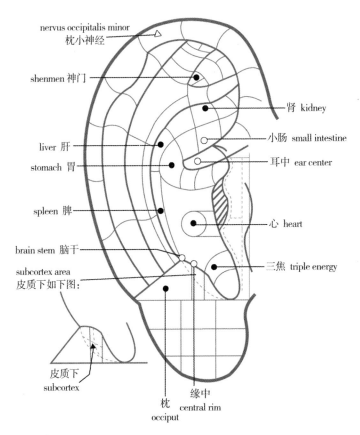

nervus occipitalis minor
枕小神经

shenmen 神门

肾 kidney

小肠 small intestine

耳中 ear center

liver 肝

stomach 胃

spleen 脾

心 heart

brain stem 脑干

subcortex area
皮质下如下图：

三焦 triple energy

皮质下
subcortex

枕
occiput

缘中
central rim

●主穴

心、神门、肝、枕、胃、肾、皮质下、脾、三焦

○配穴

小肠、枕小神经、脑干、缘中、耳中

重症肌无力
Myasthenia Gravis

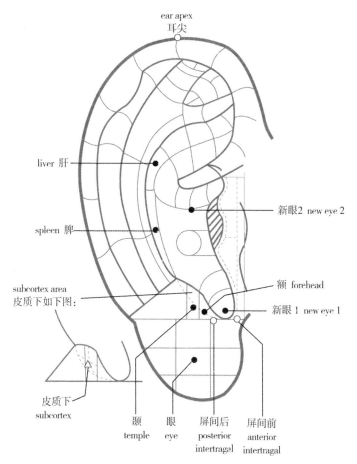

● **主穴**

肝、眼、脾、颞、额、新眼 1、新眼 2

○ **配穴**

皮质下、耳尖、屏间前、屏间后

多汗症
Hyperhidrosis

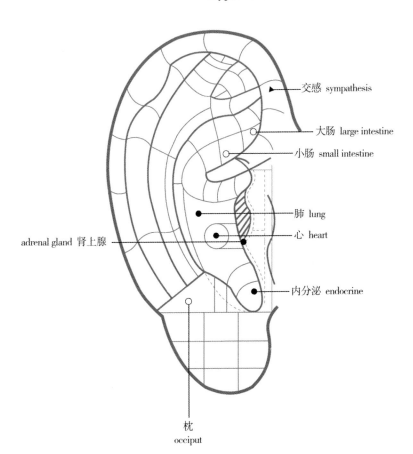

交感 sympathesis

大肠 large intestine

小肠 small intestine

肺 lung

心 heart

adrenal gland 肾上腺

内分泌 endocrine

枕
occiput

●主穴

心、肺、内分泌、交感、肾上腺

○配穴

小肠、大肠、枕

108

甲状腺功能亢进
Hyperthyrosis

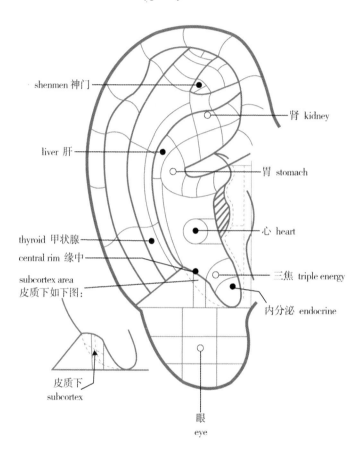

shenmen 神门

肾 kidney

liver 肝

胃 stomach

thyroid 甲状腺

心 heart

central rim 缘中

subcortex area
皮质下如下图:

三焦 triple energy

内分泌 endocrine

皮质下
subcortex

眼
eye

●主穴

肝、内分泌、缘中、神门、皮质下、甲状腺、心

○配穴

三焦、肾、胃、眼

三叉神经痛
Trigeminal Neuralgia

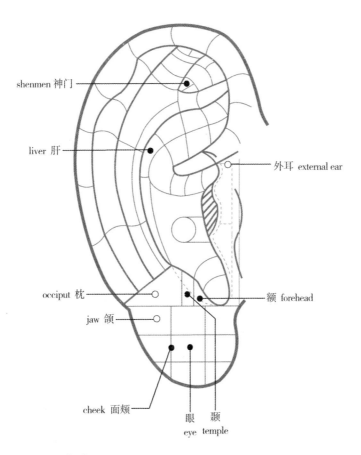

shenmen 神门

liver 肝

外耳 external ear

occiput 枕

额 forehead

jaw 颌

cheek 面颊

眼　颞
eye temple

●主穴

额、颞、面颊、肝、神门

○配穴

枕、眼、外耳、颌

肋间神经痛
Intercostal Neuralgia

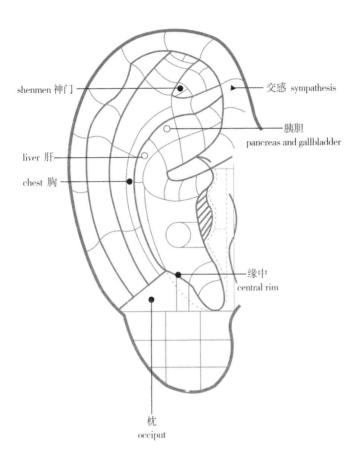

shenmen 神门

交感 sympathesis

胰胆
pancreas and gallbladder

liver 肝

chest 胸

缘中
central rim

枕
occiput

●**主穴**

缘中、神门、交感、胸、枕

○**配穴**

肝、胰胆

智力低下
Mental Retardation

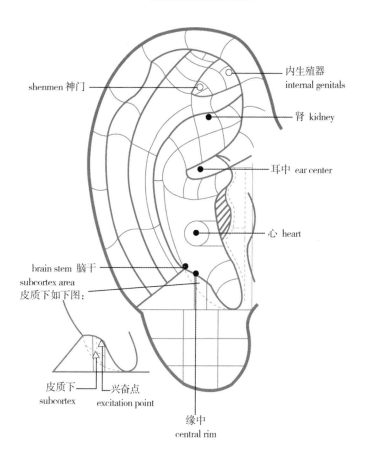

shenmen 神门

内生殖器
internal genitals

肾 kidney

耳中 ear center

心 heart

brain stem 脑干
subcortex area
皮质下如下图：

皮质下
subcortex

兴奋点
excitation point

缘中
central rim

●主穴

心、肾、耳中、脑干、缘中

○配穴

皮质下、内生殖器、神门、兴奋点

梅尼埃病
Meniere's disease

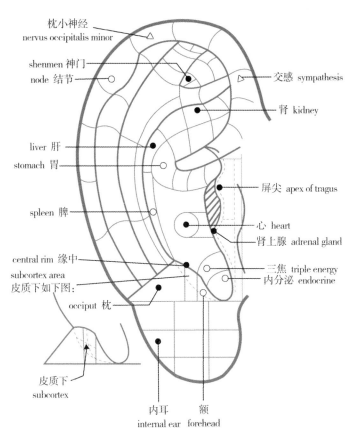

枕小神经
nervus occipitalis minor

shenmen 神门
node 结节

交感 sympathesis

肾 kidney

liver 肝
stomach 胃

屏尖 apex of tragus

spleen 脾

心 heart
肾上腺 adrenal gland

central rim 缘中
subcortex area
皮质下如下图：

三焦 triple energy
内分泌 endocrine

occiput 枕

皮质下
subcortex

内耳　　额
internal ear　forehead

●主穴

肾、神门、内耳、皮质下、枕、缘中、心、肝、肾上腺、屏尖

○配穴

枕小神经、三焦、内分泌、胃、额、交感、结节、脾

113

注意缺陷障碍
Attention Deficit Hyperactivity Disorder

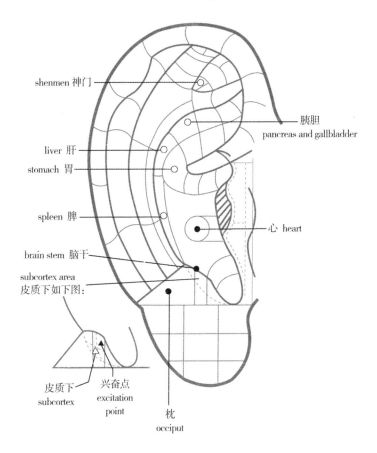

shenmen 神门

胰胆
pancreas and gallbladder

liver 肝
stomach 胃

spleen 脾

心 heart

brain stem 脑干

subcortex area
皮质下如下图：

皮质下
subcortex

兴奋点
excitation
point

枕
occiput

●主穴

心、脑干、枕、兴奋点

○配穴

神门、胰胆、肝、胃、脾、皮质下

胸痛
Chest Pain

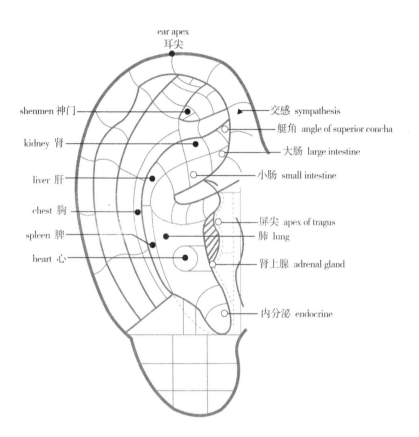

●**主穴**

心、肺、肝、胸、脾、肾、交感、神门、耳尖

○**配穴**

大肠、小肠、肾上腺、屏尖、艇角、内分泌

遗尿
Enuresis

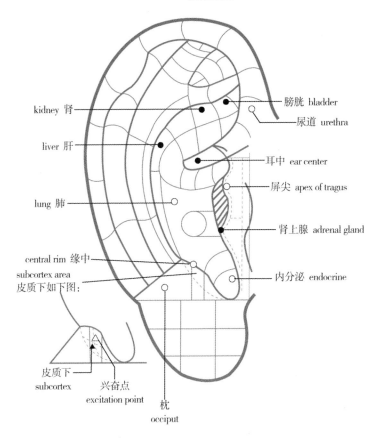

kidney 肾

liver 肝

lung 肺

central rim 缘中
subcortex area
皮质下如下图:

皮质下
subcortex

兴奋点
excitation point

膀胱 bladder

尿道 urethra

耳中 ear center

屏尖 apex of tragus

肾上腺 adrenal gland

内分泌 endocrine

枕
occiput

●主穴

肾、膀胱、肝、耳中、皮质下、肾上腺

○配穴

内分泌、缘中、尿道、兴奋点、屏尖、肺、枕

尿频
Frequent Urination

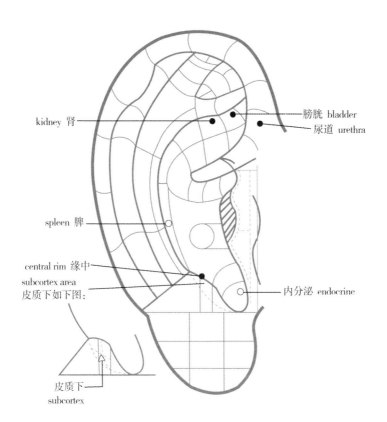

kidney 肾

膀胱 bladder
尿道 urethra

spleen 脾

central rim 缘中
subcortex area
皮质下如下图:

内分泌 endocrine

皮质下
subcortex

●主穴

肾、膀胱、缘中、尿道

○配穴

脾、内分泌、皮质下

膀胱炎
Cystitis

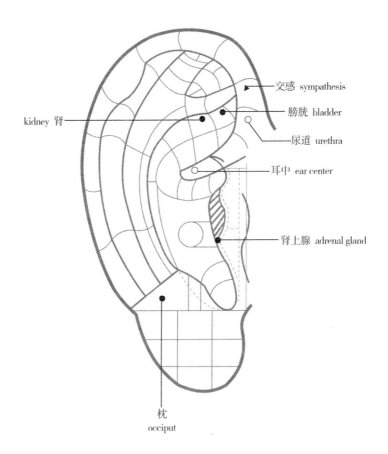

kidney 肾

交感 sympathesis

膀胱 bladder

尿道 urethra

耳中 ear center

肾上腺 adrenal gland

枕
occiput

●主穴

肾、膀胱、交感、枕、肾上腺

○配穴

尿道、耳中

肾盂肾炎
Pyelonephritis

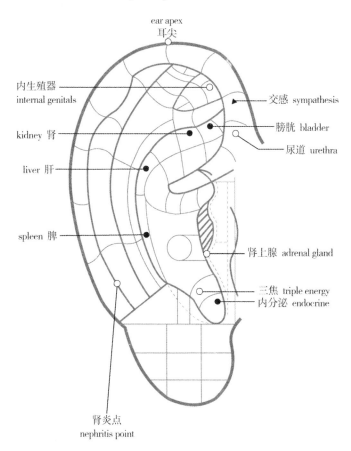

ear apex
耳尖

内生殖器
internal genitals

交感 sympathesis

kidney 肾

膀胱 bladder

尿道 urethra

liver 肝

spleen 脾

肾上腺 adrenal gland

三焦 triple energy
内分泌 endocrine

肾炎点
nephritis point

●主穴

肾、膀胱、交感、内分泌、脾、肝

○配穴

内生殖器、肾上腺、肾炎点、尿道、三焦、耳尖

急性肾炎
Acute Nephritis

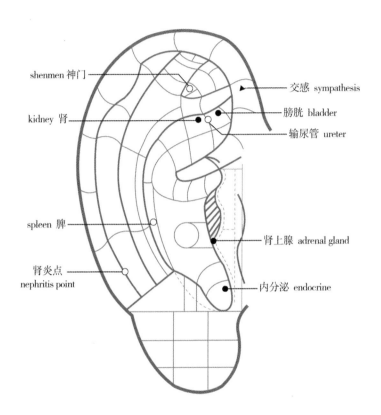

shenmen 神门

kidney 肾

spleen 脾

肾炎点
nephritis point

交感 sympathesis

膀胱 bladder

输尿管 ureter

肾上腺 adrenal gland

内分泌 endocrine

●主穴

肾、交感、膀胱、内分泌、肾上腺

○配穴

输尿管、脾、神门、肾炎点

阳痿
Impotence

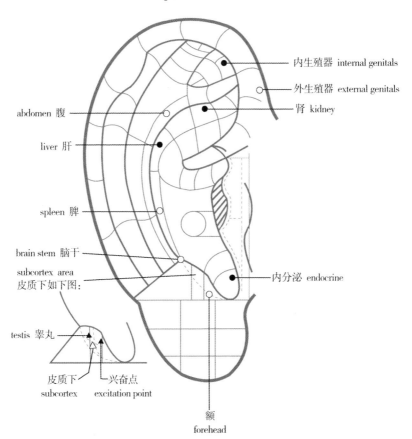

内生殖器 internal genitals

外生殖器 external genitals

肾 kidney

abdomen 腹

liver 肝

spleen 脾

brain stem 脑干

subcortex area
皮质下如下图：

内分泌 endocrine

testis 睾丸

皮质下　　　兴奋点
subcortex　excitation point

额
forehead

●主穴

内生殖器、内分泌、肝、肾、兴奋点、睾丸

○配穴

外生殖器、脾、脑干、皮质下、腹、额

睾丸炎
Orchitis

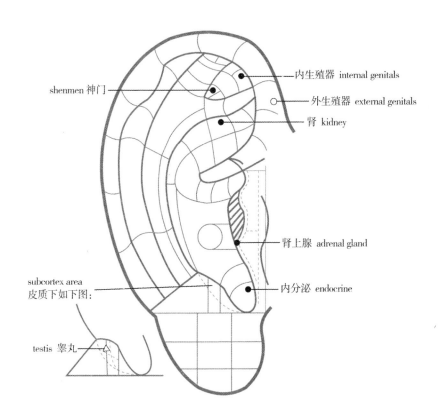

shenmen 神门

内生殖器 internal genitals

外生殖器 external genitals

肾 kidney

肾上腺 adrenal gland

内分泌 endocrine

subcortex area
皮质下如下图：

testis 睾丸

●主穴

内生殖器、内分泌、神门、肾、肾上腺

○配穴

外生殖器、睾丸

早泄
Prospermia

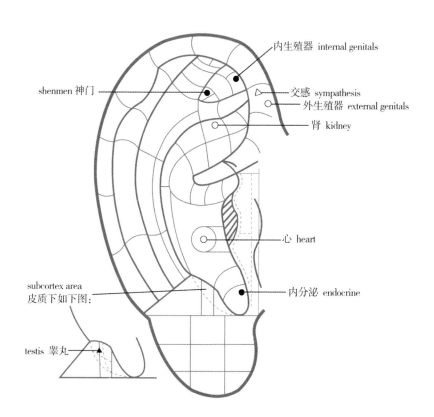

内生殖器 internal genitals

shenmen 神门

交感 sympathesis

外生殖器 external genitals

肾 kidney

心 heart

subcortex area
皮质下如下图：

内分泌 endocrine

testis 睾丸

●主穴

内生殖器、内分泌、神门、睾丸

○配穴

外生殖器、心、肾、交感

前列腺炎
Prostatitis

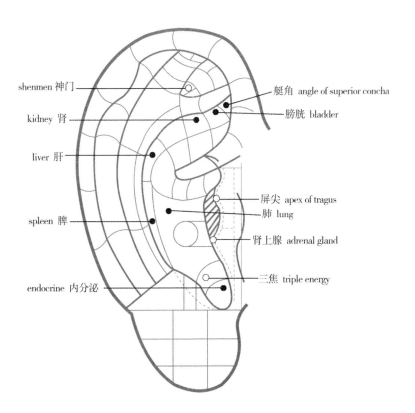

shenmen 神门

kidney 肾

liver 肝

spleen 脾

endocrine 内分泌

艇角 angle of superior concha

膀胱 bladder

屏尖 apex of tragus

肺 lung

肾上腺 adrenal gland

三焦 triple energy

●主穴

艇角、膀胱、肾、内分泌、肝、脾、肺

○配穴

肾上腺、三焦、神门、屏尖

遗精
Seminal Emission

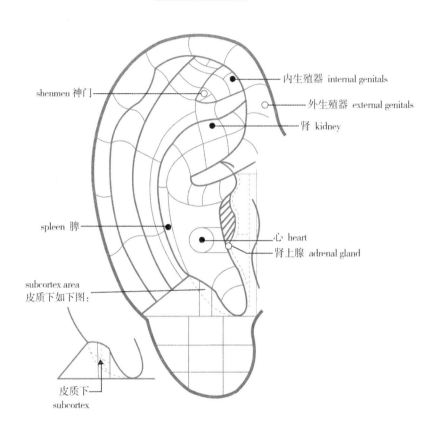

shenmen 神门

内生殖器 internal genitals

外生殖器 external genitals

肾 kidney

spleen 脾

心 heart

肾上腺 adrenal gland

subcortex area
皮质下如下图:

皮质下
subcortex

●主穴

肾、心、脾、皮质下、内生殖器

○配穴

外生殖器、神门、肾上腺

泌尿系结石
Urinary Calculi

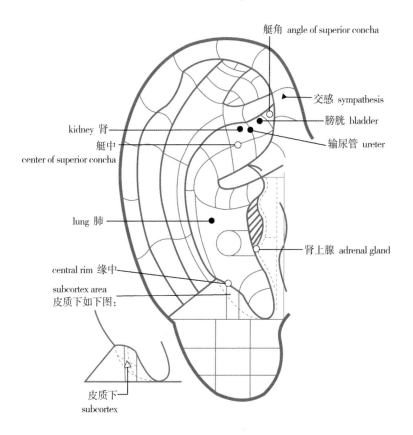

艇角 angle of superior concha

交感 sympathesis

膀胱 bladder

kidney 肾

输尿管 ureter

艇中
center of superior concha

lung 肺

肾上腺 adrenal gland

central rim 缘中

subcortex area
皮质下如下图：

皮质下
subcortex

●主穴

肺、肾、输尿管、膀胱、交感

○配穴

皮质下、缘中、肾上腺、艇中、艇角

男性不育症
Male Infertility

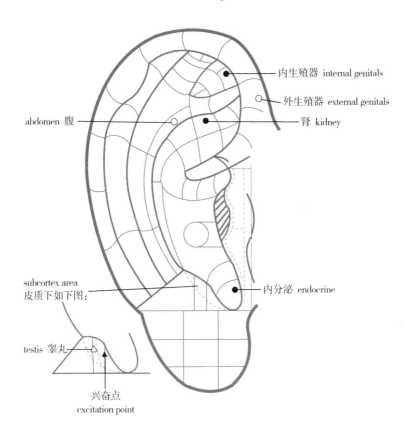

内生殖器 internal genitals
外生殖器 external genitals
abdomen 腹
肾 kidney
subcortex area
皮质下如下图：
内分泌 endocrine
testis 睾丸
兴奋点
excitation point

●主穴

肾、内生殖器、内分泌、兴奋点

○配穴

外生殖器、睾丸、腹

127

女性不孕症
Female Infertility

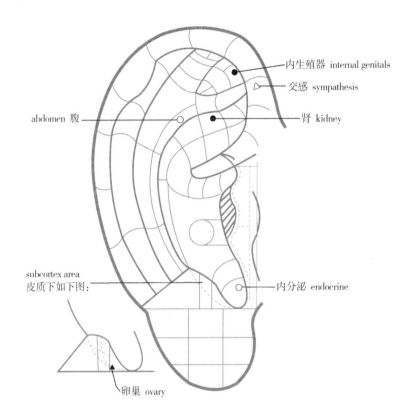

abdomen 腹

内生殖器 internal genitals

交感 sympathesis

肾 kidney

subcortex area
皮质下如下图：

内分泌 endocrine

卵巢 ovary

●主穴

内生殖器、卵巢、肾

○配穴

内分泌、交感、腹

尿道炎
Urethritis

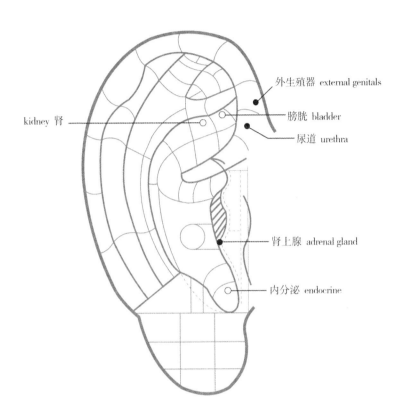

外生殖器 external genitals

膀胱 bladder

尿道 urethra

kidney 肾

肾上腺 adrenal gland

内分泌 endocrine

●主穴

外生殖器、尿道、肾上腺

○配穴

肾、膀胱、内分泌

水肿
Edema

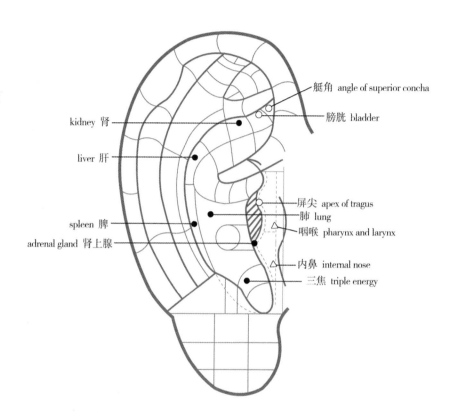

艇角 angle of superior concha

膀胱 bladder

kidney 肾

liver 肝

屏尖 apex of tragus

肺 lung

咽喉 pharynx and larynx

spleen 脾

adrenal gland 肾上腺

内鼻 internal nose

三焦 triple energy

●主穴

肾、肺、肝、脾、三焦、肾上腺

○配穴

膀胱、艇角、内鼻、咽喉、屏尖

颈椎病
Cervical Spondylosis

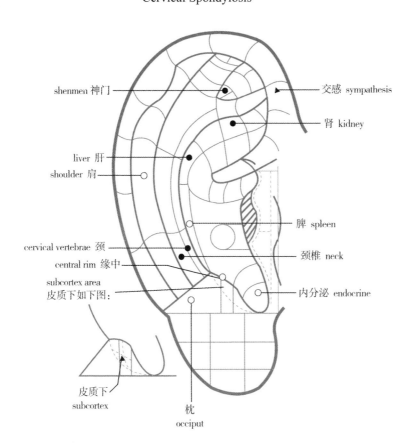

shenmen 神门

交感 sympathesis

肾 kidney

liver 肝

shoulder 肩

脾 spleen

cervical vertebrae 颈

颈椎 neck

central rim 缘中

subcortex area
皮质下如下图：

内分泌 endocrine

皮质下
subcortex

枕
occiput

●主穴

颈、颈椎、肝、肾、神门、交感、皮质下

○配穴

枕、肩、缘中、脾、内分泌

坐骨神经痛
Sciatica

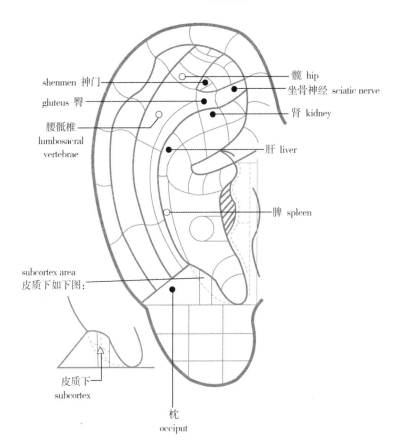

shenmen 神门

gluteus 臀

腰骶椎
lumbosacral
vertebrae

髋 hip
坐骨神经 sciatic nerve
肾 kidney

肝 liver

脾 spleen

subcortex area
皮质下如下图：

皮质下
subcortex

枕
occiput

●主穴

坐骨神经、神门、肝、肾、枕、臀

○配穴

皮质下、腰骶椎、髋、脾

落枕

Stiff Neck

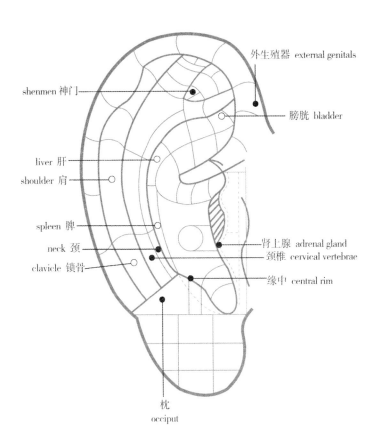

shenmen 神门

外生殖器 external genitals

膀胱 bladder

liver 肝

shoulder 肩

spleen 脾

neck 颈

clavicle 锁骨

肾上腺 adrenal gland
颈椎 cervical vertebrae

缘中 central rim

枕
occiput

●主穴

颈、颈椎、枕、缘中、神门、外生殖器、肾上腺

○配穴

肝、脾、锁骨、肩、膀胱

肩关节周围炎
Periarthritis of Shoulder

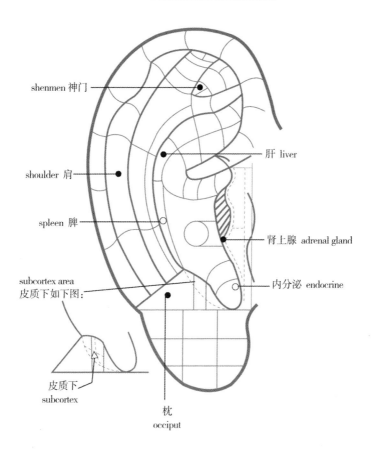

shenmen 神门

肝 liver

shoulder 肩

spleen 脾

肾上腺 adrenal gland

subcortex area
皮质下如下图:

内分泌 endocrine

皮质下
subcortex

枕
occiput

●主穴

肩、枕、神门、肾上腺、肝

○配穴

脾、内分泌、皮质下

急性腰扭伤
Acute Lumbar Sprain

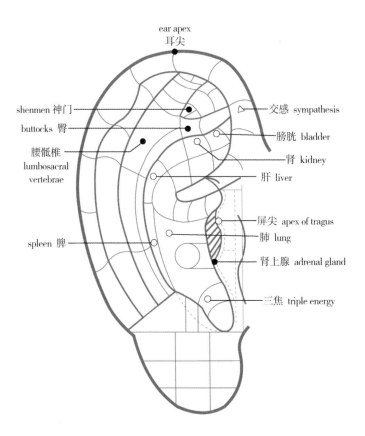

● **主穴**

耳尖、神门、腰骶椎、肾上腺、臀

○ **配穴**

肾、交感、肝、膀胱、屏尖、肺、脾、三焦

痔疮
Hemorrhoid

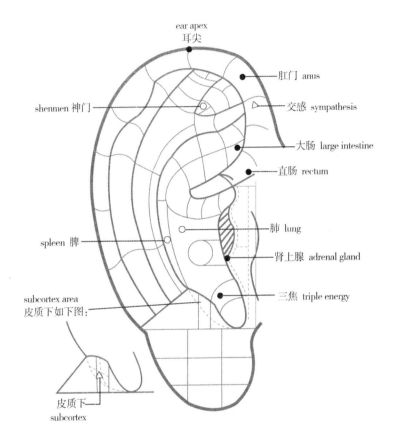

ear apex
耳尖

肛门 anus

shenmen 神门

交感 sympathesis

大肠 large intestine

直肠 rectum

肺 lung

spleen 脾

肾上腺 adrenal gland

三焦 triple energy

subcortex area
皮质下如下图：

皮质下
subcortex

●主穴

直肠、大肠、肛门、肾上腺、耳尖、三焦

○配穴

脾、神门、皮质下、交感、肺

痹证
Bi syndrome

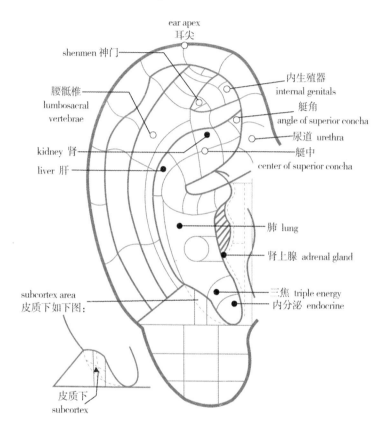

●主穴

肾、肺、肝、三焦、肾上腺、内分泌、皮质下

○配穴

艇角、尿道、耳尖、神门、内生殖器、艇中、腰骶椎

带下病
Morbid Leukorrhea

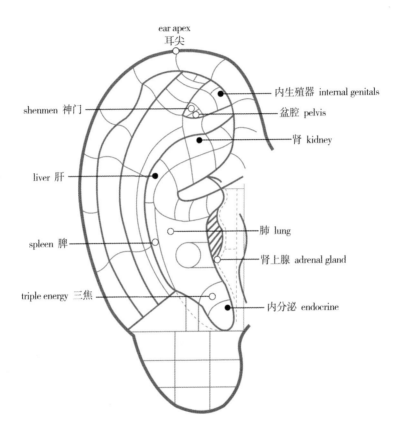

ear apex
耳尖

内生殖器 internal genitals

shenmen 神门

盆腔 pelvis

肾 kidney

liver 肝

肺 lung

spleen 脾

肾上腺 adrenal gland

triple energy 三焦

内分泌 endocrine

●主穴

内生殖器、肝、肾、内分泌

○配穴

三焦、脾、神门、肾上腺、肺、盆腔、耳尖

子宫脱垂
Hysteroptosis

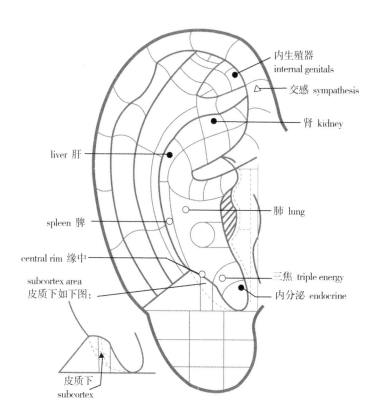

内生殖器
internal genitals

交感 sympathesis

肾 kidney

liver 肝

肺 lung

spleen 脾

central rim 缘中

subcortex area
皮质下如下图：

三焦 triple energy

内分泌 endocrine

皮质下
subcortex

●主穴

内生殖器、皮质下、肝、肾、内分泌

○配穴

三焦、交感、脾、肺、缘中

绝经期综合征
Menopausal Syndrome

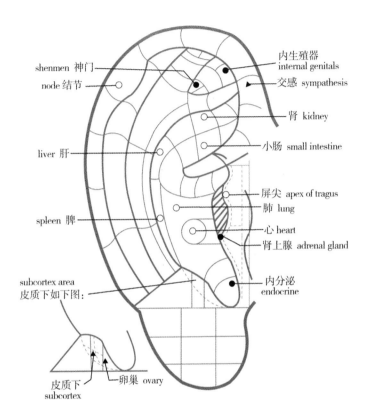

shenmen 神门
node 结节
liver 肝
spleen 脾
subcortex area
皮质下如下图：

内生殖器 internal genitals
交感 sympathesis
肾 kidney
小肠 small intestine
屏尖 apex of tragus
肺 lung
心 heart
肾上腺 adrenal gland
内分泌 endocrine

皮质下 subcortex
卵巢 ovary

●主穴

内生殖器、卵巢、内分泌、神门、交感、皮质下、肾上腺

○配穴

心、小肠、肝、肾、肺、结节、脾、屏尖

痛经
Dysmenorrhea

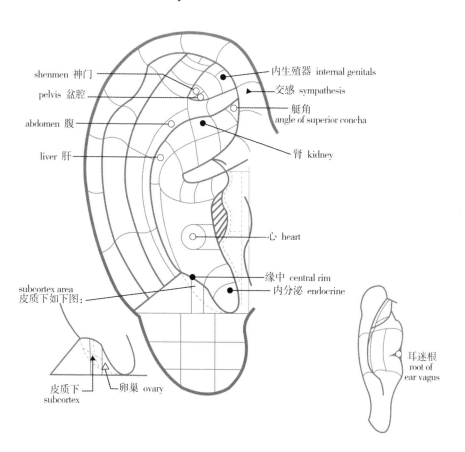

shenmen 神门
pelvis 盆腔
abdomen 腹
liver 肝
内生殖器 internal genitals
交感 sympathesis
艇角 angle of superior concha
肾 kidney
心 heart
缘中 central rim
内分泌 endocrine
subcortex area 皮质下如下图：
皮质下 subcortex
卵巢 ovary
耳迷根 root of ear vagus

●主穴

内生殖器、内分泌、交感、肾、缘中、皮质下

○配穴

卵巢、腹、神门、耳迷根、肝、心、盆腔、艇角

141

月经不调
Irregular Menstruation

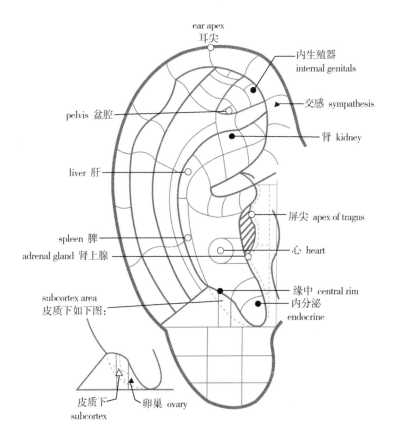

ear apex 耳尖

内生殖器 internal genitals

交感 sympathesis

pelvis 盆腔

肾 kidney

liver 肝

屏尖 apex of tragus

spleen 脾

adrenal gland 肾上腺

心 heart

subcortex area 皮质下如下图：

缘中 central rim

内分泌 endocrine

皮质下 subcortex

卵巢 ovary

●主穴

内生殖器、内分泌、交感、肾、缘中、卵巢

○配穴

心、肝、脾、耳尖、皮质下、盆腔、肾上腺、屏尖

闭经
Amenorrhea

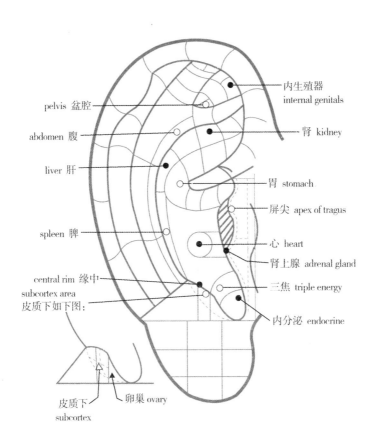

内生殖器 internal genitals
pelvis 盆腔
abdomen 腹
肾 kidney
liver 肝
胃 stomach
屏尖 apex of tragus
spleen 脾
心 heart
肾上腺 adrenal gland
central rim 缘中
subcortex area 皮质下如下图：
三焦 triple energy
内分泌 endocrine
皮质下 subcortex
卵巢 ovary

●主穴

内生殖器、内分泌、肝、肾、卵巢、心、缘中、肾上腺

○配穴

皮质下、脾、三焦、胃、屏尖、盆腔、腹

功能性子宫出血
Functional Uterine Bleeding

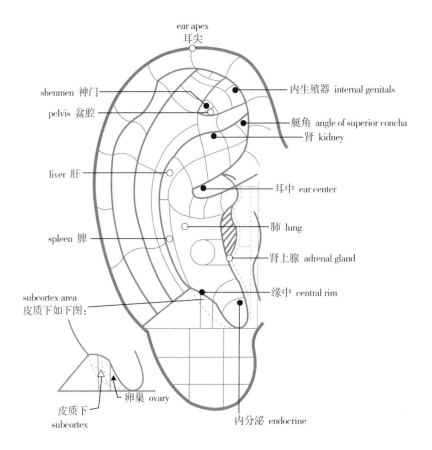

●主穴

内生殖器、艇角、缘中、肾、内分泌、神门、卵巢、耳中

○配穴

皮质下、肾上腺、肝、脾、肺、耳尖、盆腔

慢性盆腔炎
Chronic Pelvic Inflammation Disease

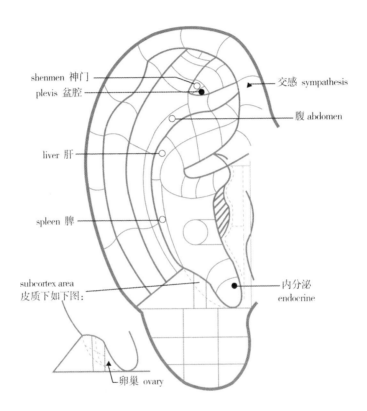

● **主穴**

内分泌、盆腔、卵巢、交感

○ **配穴**

腹、神门、脾、肝

产后宫缩痛
Afterpains

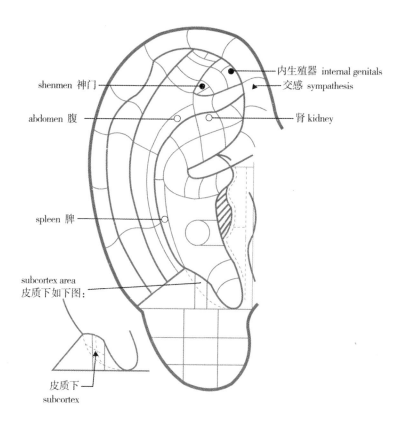

内生殖器 internal genitals
交感 sympathesis
shenmen 神门
肾 kidney
abdomen 腹
spleen 脾
subcortex area
皮质下如下图:
皮质下
subcortex

●主穴

内生殖器、交感、神门、皮质下

○配穴

腹、肾、脾

146

月经过多
Menorrhagia

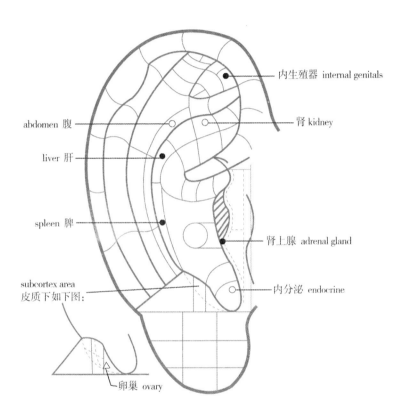

内生殖器 internal genitals

肾 kidney

abdomen 腹

liver 肝

spleen 脾

肾上腺 adrenal gland

subcortex area
皮质下如下图：

内分泌 endocrine

卵巢 ovary

●主穴

肾上腺、肝、脾、内生殖器

○配穴

肾、内分泌、卵巢、腹

乳腺增生
Hyperplasia of Mammary Glands

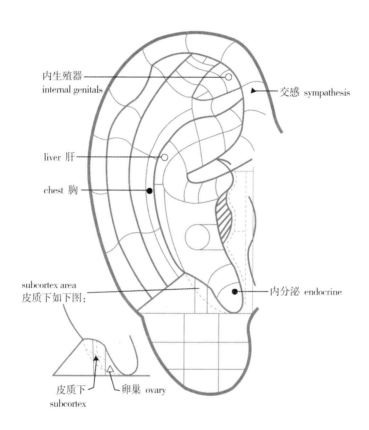

内生殖器
internal genitals

交感 sympathesis

liver 肝

chest 胸

subcortex area
皮质下如下图:

内分泌 endocrine

皮质下
subcortex

卵巢 ovary

●主穴

内分泌、皮质下、交感、胸

○配穴

卵巢、肝、内生殖器

习惯性流产
Habitual Abortion

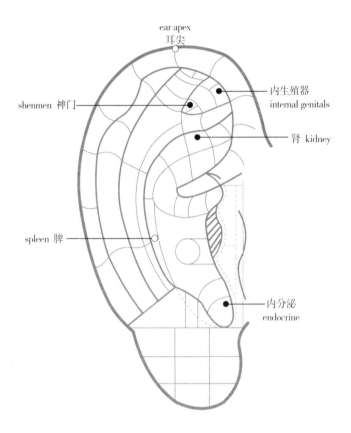

●主穴

内生殖器、肾、内分泌、神门

○配穴

脾、耳尖

妊娠恶阻
Hyperemesis Gravidarum

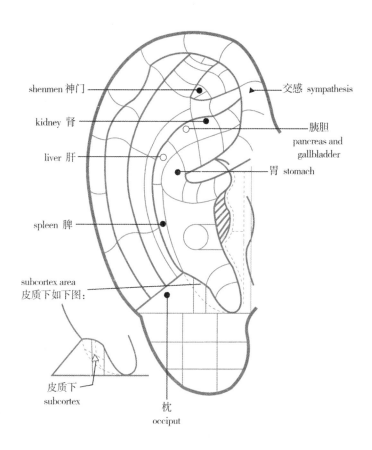

shenmen 神门

kidney 肾

liver 肝

spleen 脾

subcortex area
皮质下如下图：

皮质下
subcortex

交感 sympathesis

胰胆
pancreas and
gallbladder

胃 stomach

枕
occiput

●**主穴**

脾、胃、神门、枕、交感、肾

○**配穴**

肝、胰胆、皮质下

缺乳
Hypogalactia

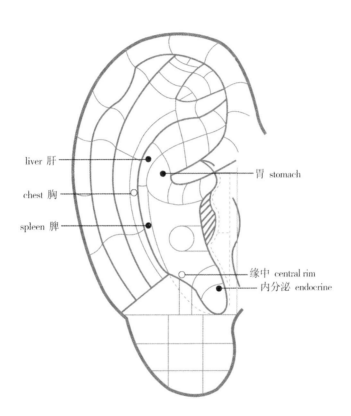

liver 肝

chest 胸

spleen 脾

胃 stomach

缘中 central rim

内分泌 endocrine

●主穴

脾、胃、内分泌、肝

○配穴

缘中、胸

胎位不正
Malposition of Fetus

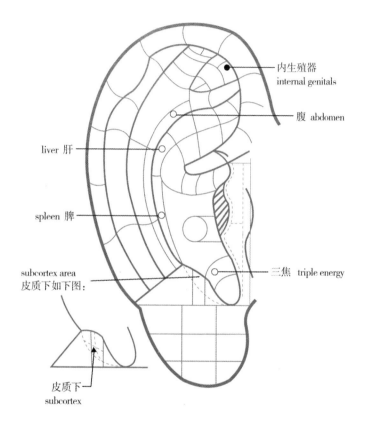

内生殖器
internal genitals

腹 abdomen

liver 肝

spleen 脾

subcortex area
皮质下如下图：

三焦 triple energy

皮质下
subcortex

●主穴

内生殖器、皮质下

○配穴

肝、脾、腹、三焦

鼻衄
Epistaxis

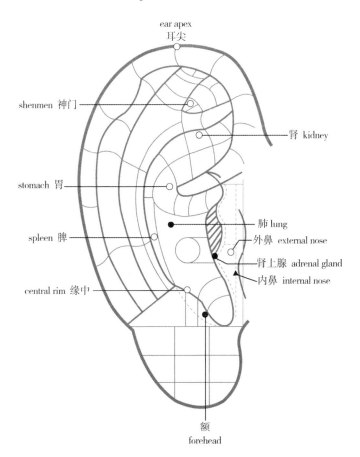

● **主穴**

肺、额、内鼻、肾上腺

○ **配穴**

外鼻、胃、缘中、神门、耳尖、脾、肾

扁桃体炎
Tonsillitis

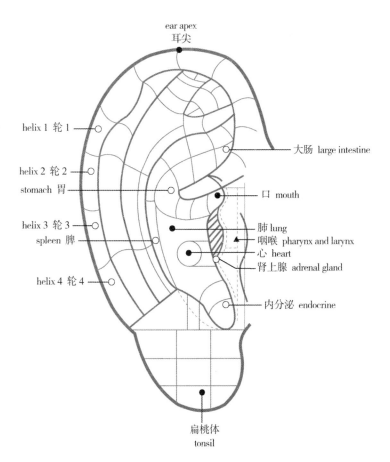

ear apex
耳尖

helix 1 轮 1

helix 2 轮 2
stomach 胃

helix 3 轮 3
spleen 脾

helix 4 轮 4

大肠 large intestine

口 mouth

肺 lung
咽喉 pharynx and larynx
心 heart
肾上腺 adrenal gland

内分泌 endocrine

扁桃体
tonsil

● 主穴

扁桃体、口、咽喉、耳尖、肺、心

○ 配穴

轮 1～轮 4、肾上腺、脾、胃、大肠、内分泌

154

过敏性鼻炎
Allergic Rhinitis

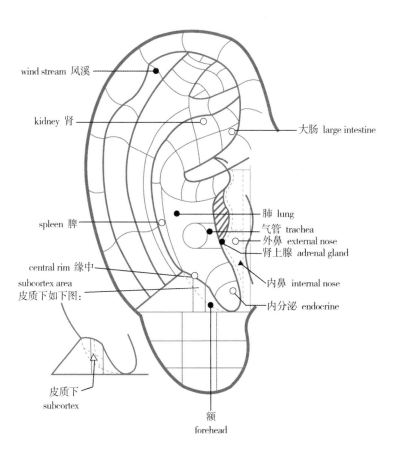

●主穴

内鼻、肾上腺、风溪、额、肺、气管

○配穴

大肠、外鼻、内分泌、脾、肾、缘中、皮质

声音嘶哑
Hoarseness

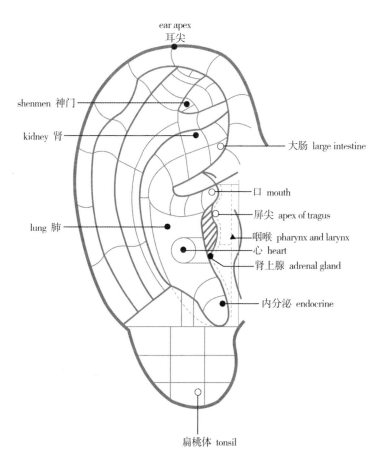

ear apex
耳尖

shenmen 神门

kidney 肾

大肠 large intestine

口 mouth

屏尖 apex of tragus

lung 肺

咽喉 pharynx and larynx

心 heart

肾上腺 adrenal gland

内分泌 endocrine

扁桃体 tonsil

●主穴

咽喉、心、肺、神门、肾、内分泌、肾上腺、耳尖

○配穴

口、扁桃体、大肠、屏尖

急、慢性咽炎
Acute and Chronic Pharyngitis

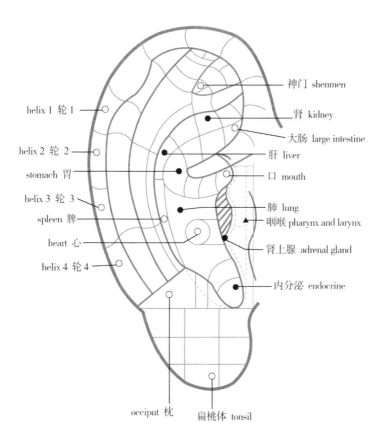

神门 shenmen

肾 kidney

大肠 large intestine

肝 liver

口 mouth

肺 lung

咽喉 pharynx and larynx

肾上腺 adrenal gland

内分泌 endocrine

helix 1 轮 1

helix 2 轮 2

stomach 胃

helix 3 轮 3

spleen 脾

heart 心

helix 4 轮 4

occiput 枕

扁桃体 tonsil

●主穴

咽喉、内分泌、肺、肾上腺、胃、肾、肝

○配穴

心、口、大肠、轮 1 ~ 轮 4、神门、枕、脾、扁桃体

面神经炎
Facial Paralysis

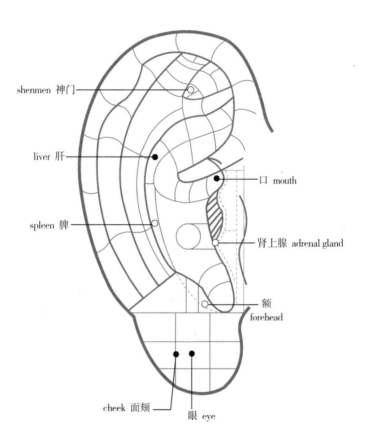

shenmen 神门

liver 肝

spleen 脾

口 mouth

肾上腺 adrenal gland

额 forehead

cheek 面颊

眼 eye

●主穴

肝、眼、面颊、口

○配穴

脾、额、神门、肾上腺

面肌痉挛
Facial Spasm

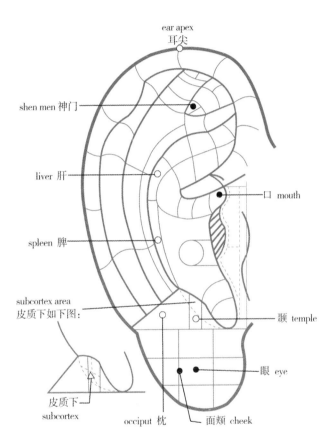

●主穴

面颊、口、神门、眼

○配穴

肝、皮质下、脾、耳尖、颞、枕

梅核气
Globus Hystericus

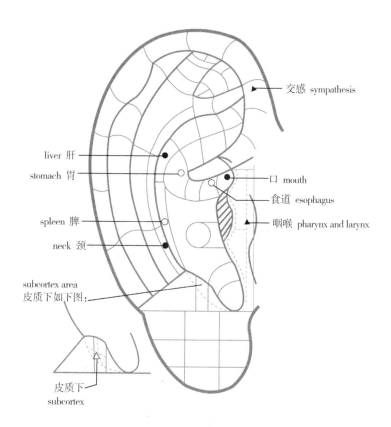

liver 肝
stomach 胃
spleen 脾
neck 颈
subcortex area
皮质下如下图：
皮质下
subcortex

交感 sympathesis
口 mouth
食道 esophagus
咽喉 pharynx and larynx

●主穴

肝、颈、咽喉、口、交感

○配穴

胃、脾、皮质下、食道

160

中耳炎
Otitis Media

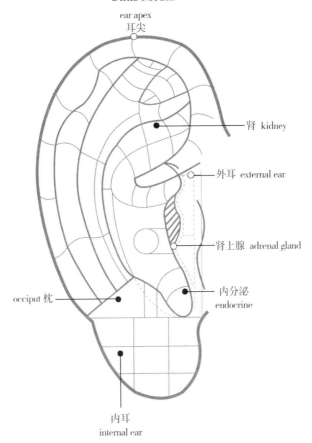

ear apex
耳尖

肾 kidney

外耳 external ear

肾上腺 adrenal gland

occiput 枕

内分泌
endocrine

内耳
internal ear

●主穴

肾、内耳、内分泌、枕

○配穴

外耳、肾上腺、耳尖

耳鸣
Tinnitus

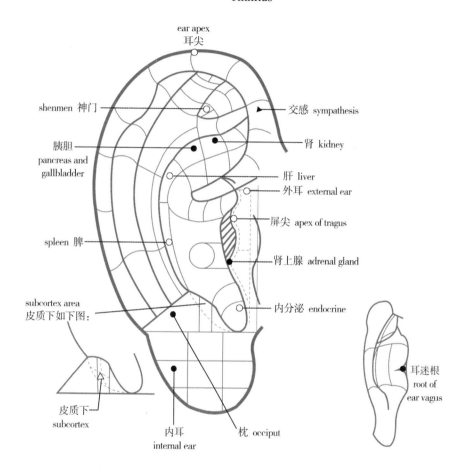

ear apex 耳尖

shenmen 神门

胰胆 pancreas and gallbladder

spleen 脾

subcortex area 皮质下如下图：

皮质下 subcortex

交感 sympathesis

肾 kidney

肝 liver

外耳 external ear

屏尖 apex of tragus

肾上腺 adrenal gland

内分泌 endocrine

内耳 internal ear

枕 occiput

耳迷根 root of ear vagus

●主穴

肾、枕、胰胆、内耳、交感、肾上腺、耳迷根

○配穴

肝、外耳、神门、耳尖、皮质下、脾、内分泌、屏尖

麦粒肿
Hordeolum

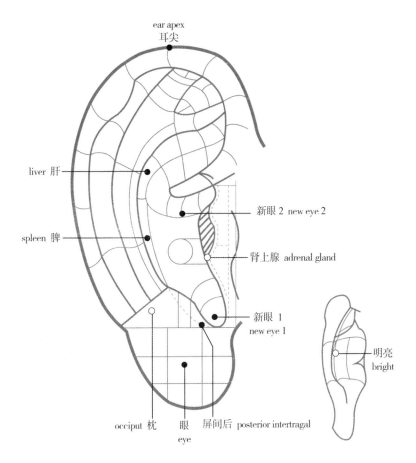

●主穴

肝、脾、眼、耳尖、新眼 1、新眼 2、屏间后

○配穴

肾上腺、枕、明亮

163

霰粒肿
Chalazion

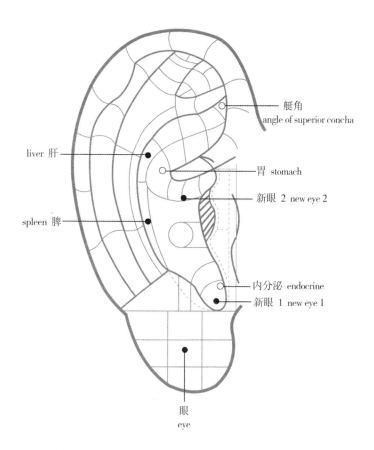

艇角
angle of superior concha

liver 肝

胃 stomach

新眼 2 new eye 2

spleen 脾

内分泌 endocrine

新眼 1 new eye 1

眼
eye

● **主穴**

肝、脾、眼、新眼 1、新眼 2

○ **配穴**

内分泌、胃、艇角

电光性眼炎

Electric Ophthalmia

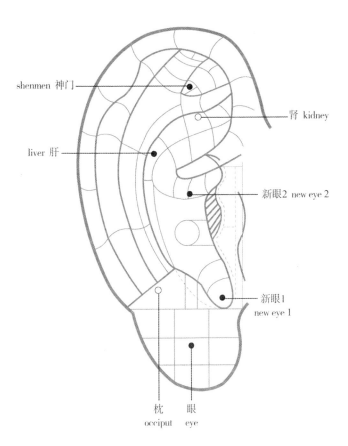

shenmen 神门

肾 kidney

liver 肝

新眼2 new eye 2

新眼1
new eye 1

枕　　眼
occiput　eye

●主穴

肝、眼、神门、新眼 1、新眼 2

○配穴

枕、肾

近视、远视、散光、弱视
Myopia,Hypermetropia,Astigmatism and Amblyopia

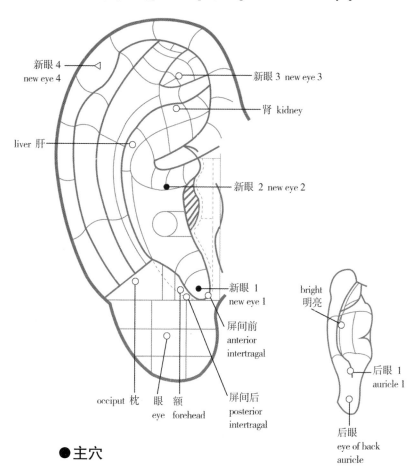

●主穴

新眼 1、新眼 2

○配穴

新眼 3、新眼 4、肝、眼、枕、肾、明亮、后眼 1、后眼、
额、屏间前、屏间后

166

青光眼
Glaucoma

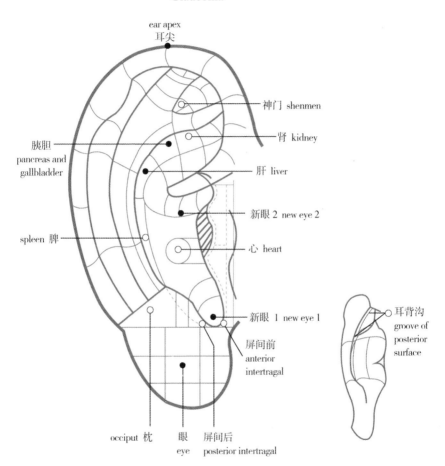

●**主穴**

眼、耳尖、新眼1、新眼2、肝、胰胆

○**配穴**

肾、心、脾、枕、神门、耳背沟、屏间前、屏间后

视神经萎缩
Optic Atrophy

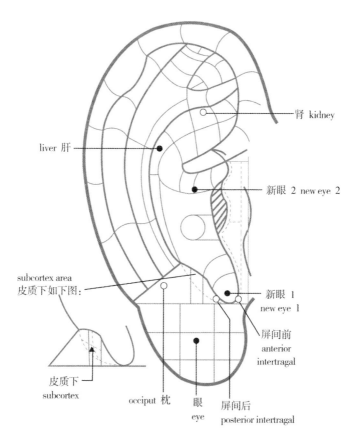

肾 kidney

liver 肝

新眼 2 new eye 2

subcortex area
皮质下如下图：

新眼 1
new eye 1

屏间前
anterior
intertragal

皮质下
subcortex

occiput 枕

眼
eye

屏间后
posterior intertragal

●主穴

眼、肝、新眼 1、新眼 2、皮质下

○配穴

肾、枕、屏间前、屏间后

168

急性结膜炎
Acute Conjunctivitis

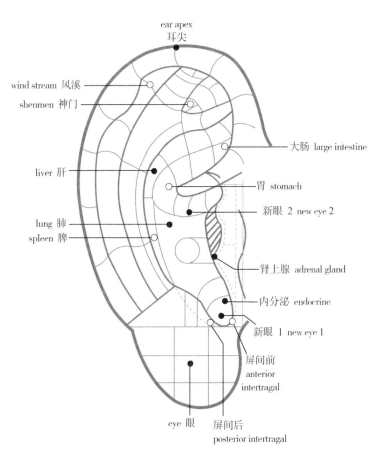

●主穴

眼、肝、新眼1、新眼2、肺、耳尖、内分泌、肾上腺

○配穴

风溪、大肠、神门、屏间前、脾、胃、屏间后

口疮
Aphtha

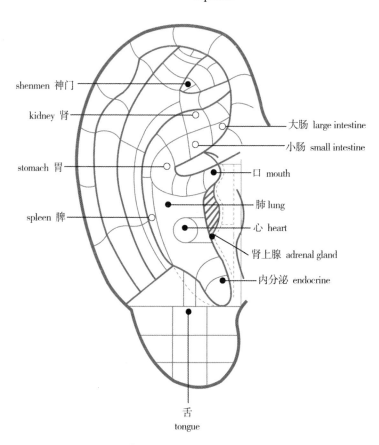

shenmen 神门

kidney 肾

大肠 large intestine

小肠 small intestine

stomach 胃

口 mouth

肺 lung

spleen 脾

心 heart

肾上腺 adrenal gland

内分泌 endocrine

舌
tongue

●主穴

心、口、内分泌、舌、肺、神门、肾上腺

○配穴

胃、脾、大肠、小肠、肾

瘙痒症
Pruritus

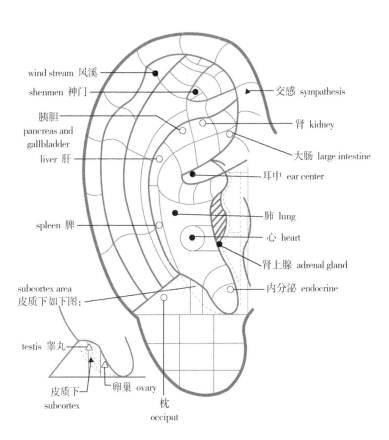

●主穴

肺、神门、皮质下、肾上腺、风溪、心、耳中、交感

○配穴

肝、脾、内分泌、胰胆、睾丸、卵巢、枕、大肠、肾

银屑病
Psoriasis

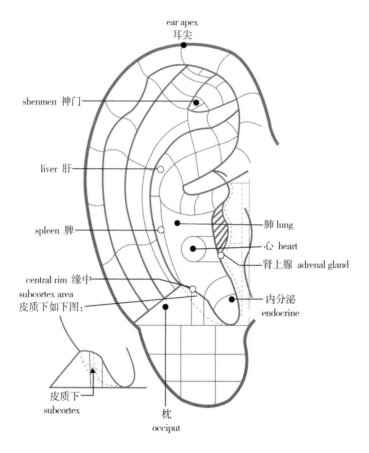

ear apex
耳尖

shenmen 神门

liver 肝

spleen 脾

肺 lung

心 heart

肾上腺 adrenal gland

central rim 缘中
subcortex area
皮质下如下图:

内分泌
endocrine

皮质下
subcortex

枕
occiput

●主穴

肺、心、内分泌、枕、耳尖、神门、皮质下

○配穴

肾上腺、肝、脾、缘中

外阴瘙痒
Pruritus Vulvae

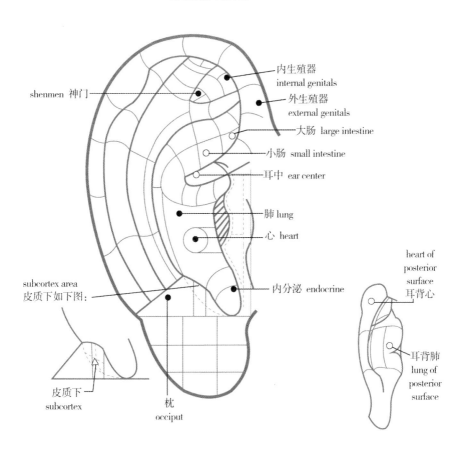

●主穴

内生殖器、外生殖器、心、神门、内分泌、枕、肺

○配穴

小肠、耳中、大肠、皮质下、耳背心、耳背肺

173

过敏性皮炎
Allergic Dermatitis

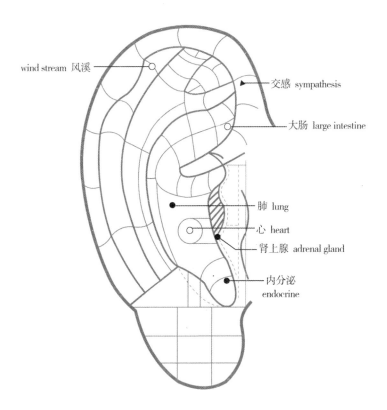

wind stream 风溪

交感 sympathesis

大肠 large intestine

肺 lung

心 heart

肾上腺 adrenal gland

内分泌
endocrine

●主穴

肺、内分泌、肾上腺、交感

○配穴

风溪、大肠、心

脂溢性皮炎
Seborrheic Dermatitis

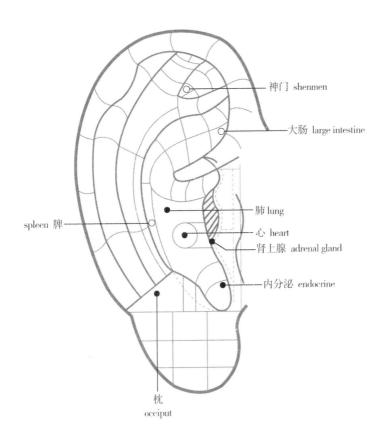

神门 shenmen

大肠 large intestine

肺 lung

心 heart

肾上腺 adrenal gland

spleen 脾

内分泌 endocrine

枕
occiput

●主穴

心、肺、内分泌、肾上腺、枕

○配穴

大肠、神门、脾

荨麻疹
Urticaria

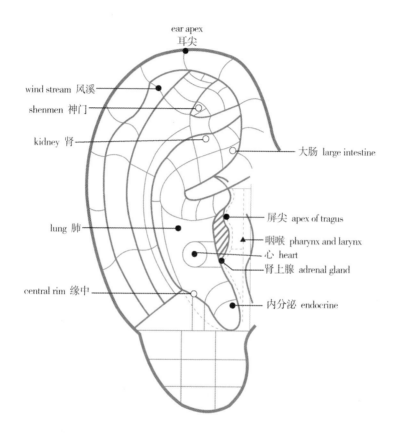

●**主穴**

肺、风溪、内分泌、肾上腺、咽喉、屏尖、耳尖、心

○**配穴**

大肠、神门、缘中、肾

硬皮病
Dermatosclerosis

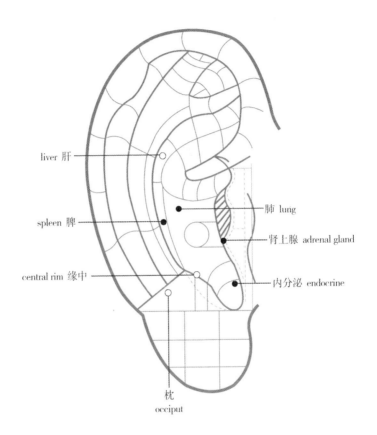

liver 肝
spleen 脾
central rim 缘中
肺 lung
肾上腺 adrenal gland
内分泌 endocrine
枕
occiput

●主穴

肺、脾、肾上腺、内分泌

○配穴

缘中、肝、枕

177

痤疮
Acne

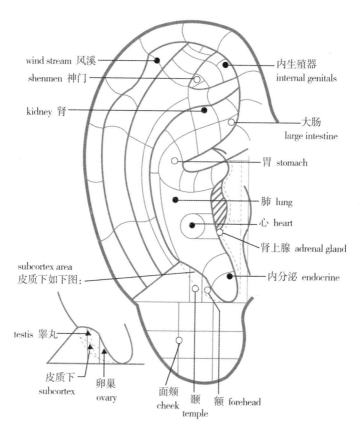

wind stream 风溪
shenmen 神门
kidney 肾
内生殖器 internal genitals
大肠 large intestine
胃 stomach
肺 lung
心 heart
肾上腺 adrenal gland
内分泌 endocrine
subcortex area 皮质下如下图:
testis 睾丸
皮质下 subcortex
卵巢 ovary
面颊 cheek
颞 temple
额 forehead

●主穴

肺、内分泌、肾、内生殖器、心、皮质下、风溪、卵巢、睾丸

○配穴

颞、额、大肠、肾上腺、面颊、神门、胃

肥胖症
Obesity

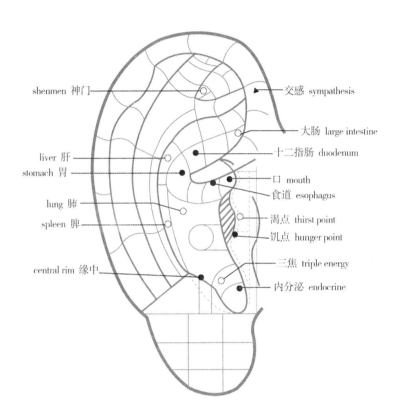

shenmen 神门

交感 sympathesis

大肠 large intestine

十二指肠 duodenum

liver 肝

stomach 胃

口 mouth

食道 esophagus

lung 肺

spleen 脾

渴点 thirst point

饥点 hunger point

central rim 缘中

三焦 triple energy

内分泌 endocrine

●主穴

口、食道、胃、十二指肠、内分泌、饥点、交感、缘中

○配穴

肺、三焦、大肠、神门、渴点、脾、肝

179

黄褐斑
Chloasma

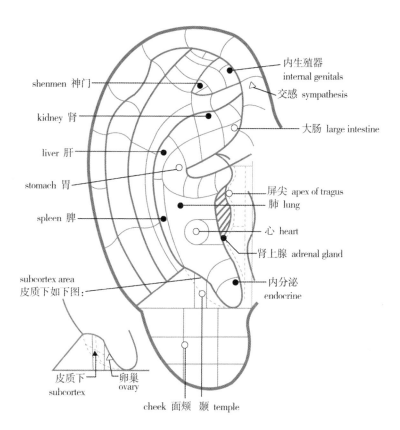

shenmen 神门

kidney 肾

liver 肝

stomach 胃

spleen 脾

subcortex area
皮质下如下图：

皮质下
subcortex
卵巢
ovary

cheek 面颊　颞 temple

内生殖器 internal genitals
交感 sympathesis
大肠 large intestine
屏尖 apex of tragus
肺 lung
心 heart
肾上腺 adrenal gland
内分泌 endocrine

●主穴

内生殖器、肝、肾、脾、内分泌、皮质下、肺、神门、肾上腺

○配穴

心、胃、大肠、卵巢、交感、面颊、颞、屏尖

脱发
Baldness

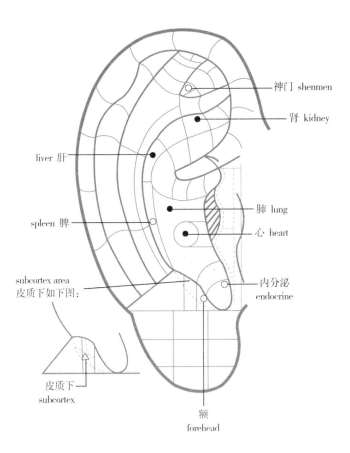

神门 shenmen

肾 kidney

liver 肝

肺 lung

spleen 脾

心 heart

subcortex area
皮质下如下图：

内分泌
endocrine

皮质下
subcortex

额
forehead

●主穴

心、肝、肾、肺

○配穴

脾、内分泌、皮质下、神门、额

181

美容
Beauty

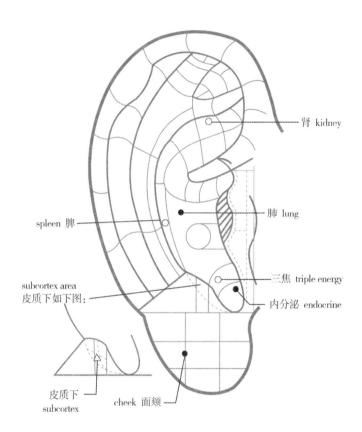

肾 kidney

肺 lung

spleen 脾

三焦 triple energy

内分泌 endocrine

subcortex area
皮质下如下图：

皮质下
subcortex

cheek 面颊

●主穴

肺、面颊、内分泌

○配穴

皮质下、脾、肾、三焦

伤风、感冒
Common Cold

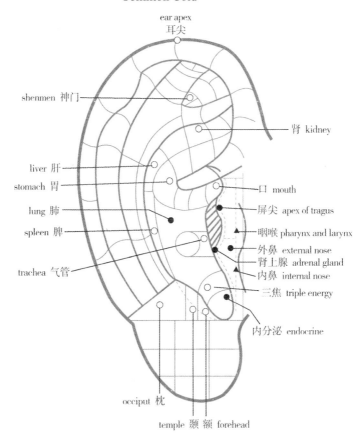

ear apex
耳尖

shenmen 神门

肾 kidney

liver 肝

stomach 胃

口 mouth

lung 肺

屏尖 apex of tragus

spleen 脾

咽喉 pharynx and larynx

外鼻 external nose

肾上腺 adrenal gland

trachea 气管

内鼻 internal nose

三焦 triple energy

内分泌 endocrine

occiput 枕

temple 颞 额 forehead

●主穴

内鼻、外鼻、肺、肾上腺、内分泌、咽喉、屏尖

○配穴

耳尖、额、神门、颞、肝、三焦、枕、口、气管、脾、胃、肾

183

糖尿病
Diabetes

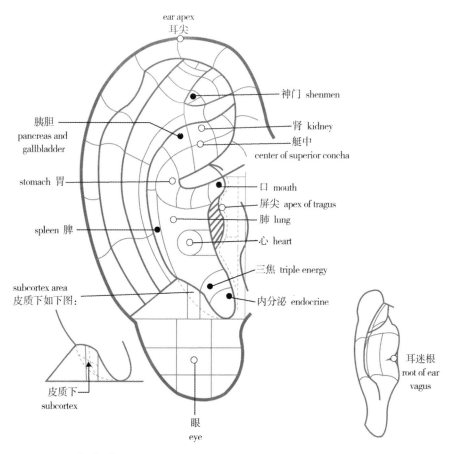

●**主穴**

胰胆、内分泌、口、神门、三焦、皮质下、脾

○**配穴**

肺、胃、肾、艇中、眼、耳迷根、心、耳尖、屏尖

雷诺病
Raynaud Disease

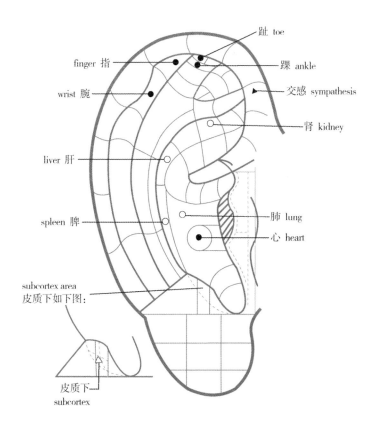

● **主穴**

心、交感、指、趾、腕、踝

○ **配穴**

肾、肝、脾、肺、皮质下

竞技综合征
Athletic Competition Syndrome

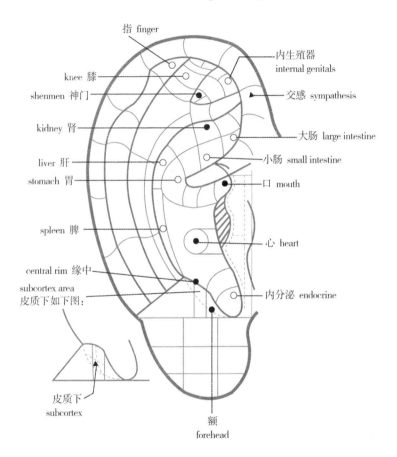

●主穴

心、肾、交感、神门、皮质下、缘中、额、口

○配穴

大肠、小肠、胃、内分泌、内生殖器、肝、脾、指、膝

戒断综合征
Withdrawal Syndrome

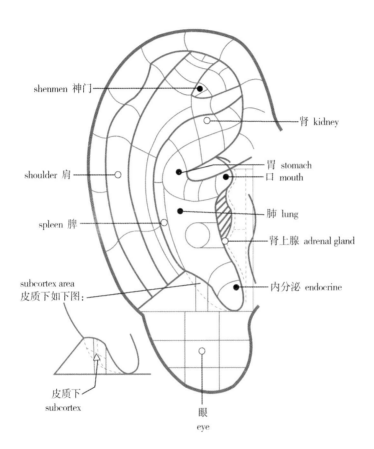

●**主穴**

肺、口、胃、神门、内分泌

○**配穴**

眼、肩、肾、脾、皮质下、肾上腺

187

晕动病
Motion Sickness

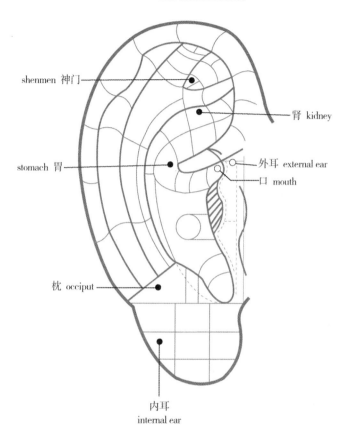

shenmen 神门

肾 kidney

stomach 胃

外耳 external ear

口 mouth

枕 occiput

内耳
internal ear

●主穴

枕、内耳、肾、神门、胃

○配穴

外耳、口

戒烟
Giving up smoking

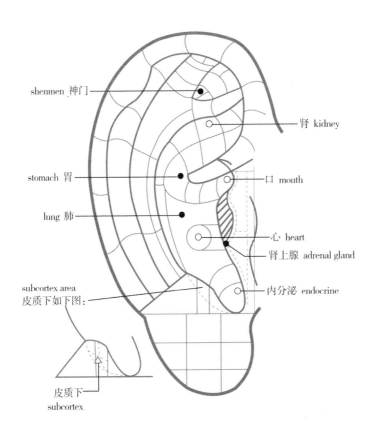

●主穴

肾上腺、肺、胃、神门

○配穴

皮质下、内分泌、心、口、肾

戒酒
Stopping Drinking

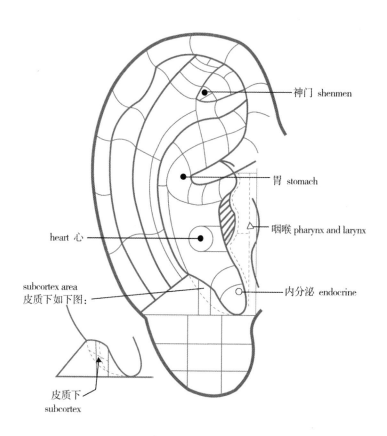

神门 shenmen

胃 stomach

咽喉 pharynx and larynx

heart 心

subcortex area
皮质下如下图:

内分泌 endocrine

皮质下
subcortex

●主穴

心、胃、神门、皮质下

○配穴

内分泌、咽喉

小儿热病
Infantile Febrile Disease

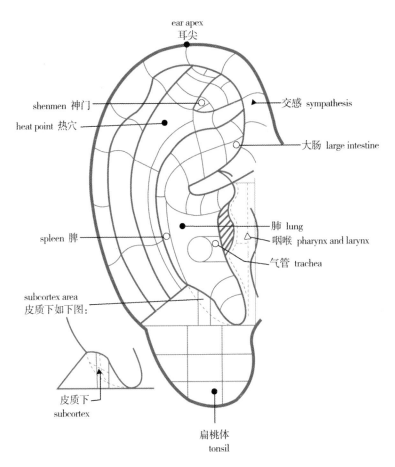

●**主穴**

肺、耳尖、交感、扁桃体、热穴、皮质下

○**配穴**

神门、气管、咽喉、脾、大肠

疲劳
Fatigue

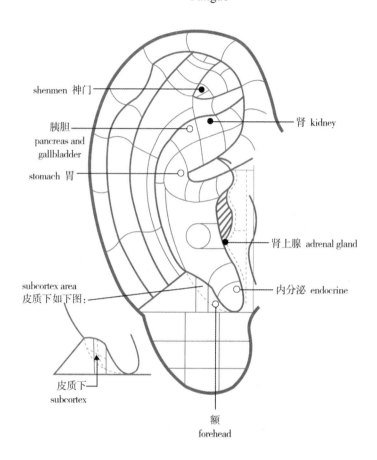

shenmen 神门

胰胆
pancreas and
gallbladder

stomach 胃

subcortex area
皮质下如下图:

皮质下
subcortex

肾 kidney

肾上腺 adrenal gland

内分泌 endocrine

额
forehead

●主穴

肾、皮质下、肾上腺、神门

○配穴

内分泌、胰胆、胃、额

耳廓解剖名称示意图（正、背面）

Anatomical nomenclature of the auricle (front and back view)

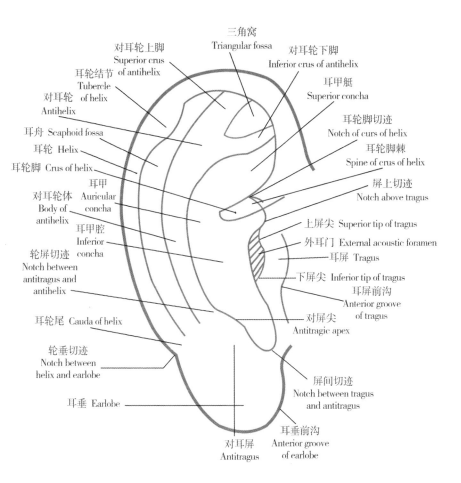

三角窝
Triangular fossa

对耳轮上脚
Superior crus
of antihelix

对耳轮下脚
Inferior crus of antihelix

耳轮结节
Tubercle
of helix

耳甲艇
Superior concha

对耳轮
Antihelix

耳轮脚切迹
Notch of curs of helix

耳舟 Scaphoid fossa

耳轮脚棘
Spine of crus of helix

耳轮 Helix

耳轮脚 Crus of helix

屏上切迹
Notch above tragus

耳甲
Auricular
concha

对耳轮体
Body of
antihelix

上屏尖 Superior tip of tragus

外耳门 External acoustic foramen

耳甲腔
Inferior
concha

耳屏 Tragus

下屏尖 Inferior tip of tragus

轮屏切迹
Notch between
antitragus and
antihelix

耳屏前沟
Anterior groove
of tragus

耳轮尾 Cauda of helix

对屏尖
Antitragic apex

轮垂切迹
Notch between
helix and earlobe

屏间切迹
Notch between tragus
and antitragus

耳垂 Earlobe

对耳屏
Antitragus

耳垂前沟
Anterior groove
of earlobe

耳廓解剖名称示意图（正、背面）

Anatomical nomenclature of the auricle (front and back view)

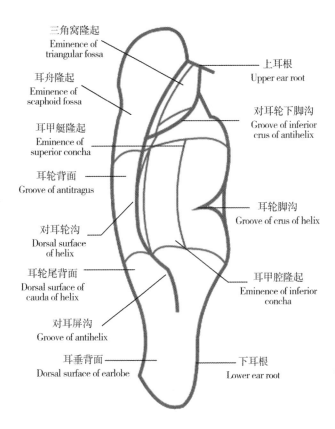

三角窝隆起
Eminence of
triangular fossa

耳舟隆起
Eminence of
scaphoid fossa

耳甲艇隆起
Eminence of
superior concha

耳轮背面
Groove of antitragus

对耳轮沟
Dorsal surface
of helix

耳轮尾背面
Dorsal surface of
cauda of helix

对耳屏沟
Groove of antihelix

耳垂背面
Dorsal surface of earlobe

上耳根
Upper ear root

对耳轮下脚沟
Groove of inferior
crus of antihelix

耳轮脚沟
Groove of crus of helix

耳甲腔隆起
Eminence of inferior
concha

下耳根
Lower ear root

病症索引

M

N

P

Q

Z

Disease Index

A

9

H

I

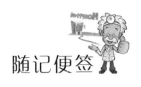

随记便签

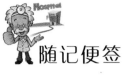

随记便签

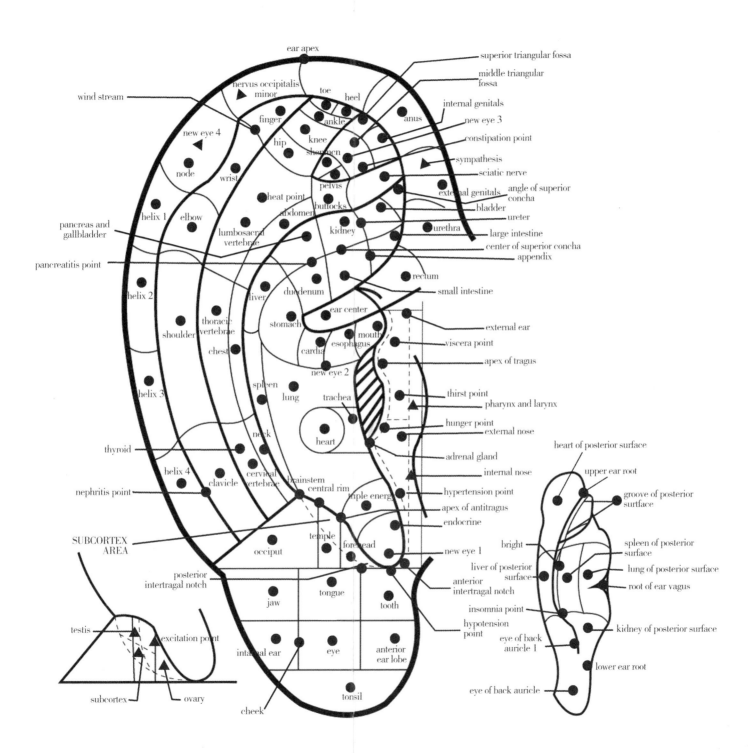

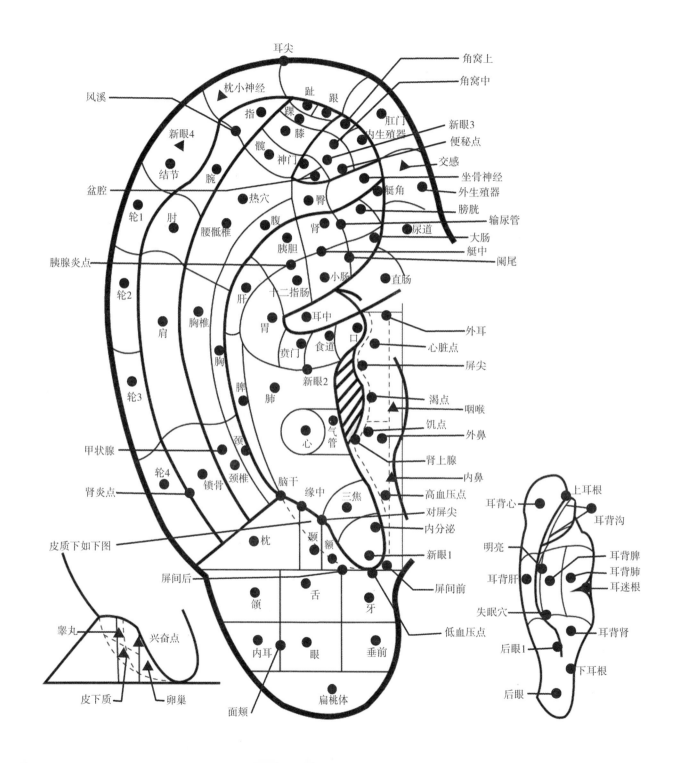